HEARTPLAN

ALSO BY MARK RUBINSTEIN, M.D.

New Choices: The Latest Options in Treating Breast Cancer (with Dennis P. Cirillo, M.D.)

The Complete Book of Cosmetic Facial Surgery (with Dennis P. Cirillo, M.D.)

The First Encounter: The Beginnings in Psychotherapy (with William A. Console, M.D., and Richard C. Simons, M.D.)

David L. Copen, M.D.,
and Mark Rubinstein, M.D.

HEART-PLAN

A Complete Program for Total Fitness of Heart & Mind

McGraw-Hill Book Company

New York　St. Louis　San Francisco　Hamburg　Mexico　Toronto

Copyright ©1987 by David L. Copen, M.D., and Mark Rubinstein, M.D. All rights reserved. Printed in the United States of America. Except as permitted under the Copyright Act of 1976, no part of this publication may be reproduced or distributed in any form or by any means or stored in a data base or retrieval system, without the prior written permission of the publisher.

123456789DOC/DOC876

ISBN 0-07-054205-8

LIBRARY OF CONGRESS CATALOGING-IN-PUBLICATION DATA

Copen, David.
   Heartplan: a complete program for total fitness of heart and mind.
   Bibliography: p.
   Includes index.
   1. Heart—Diseases—Prevention—Popular works.
2. Heart—Diseases—Psychological aspects—Popular works.   3. Stress (Psychology).
4. Type A behavior.
I. Rubenstein, Mark, 1942-   [DNLM: 1. Heart Diseases—prevention & control—popular works.
2. Stress, Psychological—prevention & control—popular works. WG 113 C7823h]
RC681.C694 1986   616.1'205   86-7433
ISBN 0-07-054205-8

BOOK DESIGN BY PATRICE FODERO

For Joshua and Harry

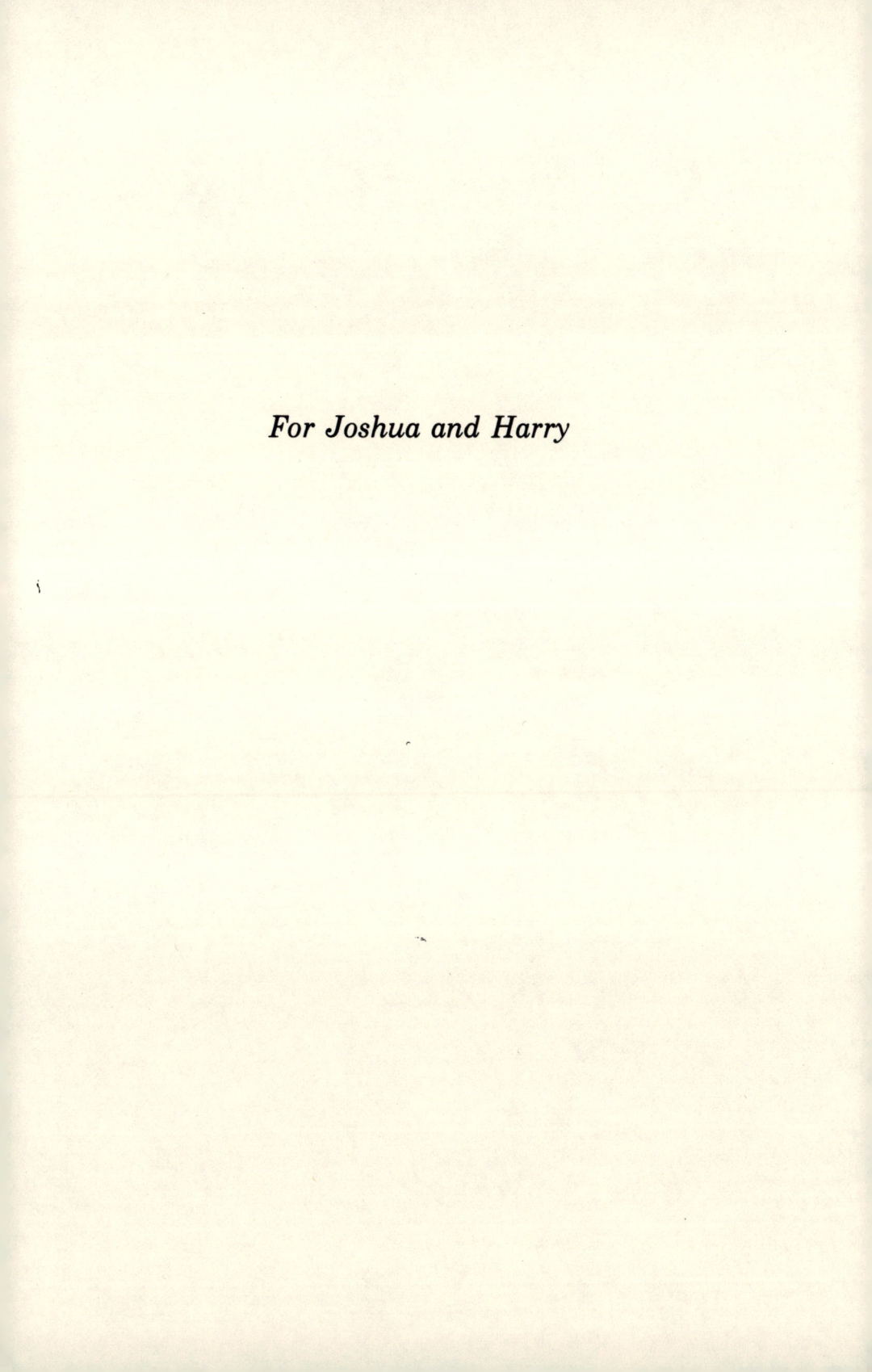

Acknowledgments

We wish to thank our wives, Claire Copen and Linda Rubinstein, for their creative input and guidance throughout every phase of this book. We also owe a debt of gratitude to Vernon Sutter, Edith Sutter, Dave Smyth, and Anne Smyth who read the manuscript and made many helpful suggestions.

David L. Copen, M.D.
Mark Rubinstein, M.D.

Contents

Introduction xi
Note to the Reader xv

PART 1: THE PROBLEM

Chapter 1: The Heart-Mind Connection 1
Chapter 2: Your Heart in Health and Disease 5
Chapter 3: The Risks: How They Affect You................... 15
Chapter 4: Know the Enemy: Stress, the Most
 Dangerous Risk.. 31
Chapter 5: The Deadly Triple Play 37
Chapter 6: Heart Attack: The Ultimate Challenge 53
Chapter 7: Beyond the CCU: Adjusting to New
 (and Not-So-Bad) Realities......................... 61

PART 2: HEARTPLAN: A STEP-BY-STEP STRATEGY FOR PHYSICAL AND EMOTIONAL WELL-BEING

Step 1: Setting New Priorities and Realistic Goals............ 71

Step 2: Decreasing Both Obvious and Invisible
          Emotional Entrapment 78
Step 3: Modifying Type A Behavior 86
Step 4: Reducing Both Large and Small Stresses 92
Step 5: Eating for Health and Pleasure 101
Step 6: All about Exercise 137
Step 7: Relaxation 145
Step 8: To Stop Smoking 149
Step 9: Your Medical Program 156

PART 3: ANYTHING ELSE YOU NEED TO KNOW

Chapter 8: Your Sex Life 169
Chapter 9: Living with a Heart Patient 173
Chapter 10: All about Heart Surgery 183
Chapter 11: The Future 195
Selected References 201
Index 207

Introduction

Heart disease is the plague of the twentieth century: Nearly 42 million Americans have cardiovascular—or heart—disease. It is our number-one killer and crippler, it costs an estimated $72.1 billion per year, and yet few people have a realistic strategy for dealing with it.*

In addition to the millions who have high blood pressure and angina pectoris chest pains, 1.5 million Americans have heart attacks every year. Of the 1 million who survive, fewer than half return to productive, satisfying lives.

Furthermore, the millions who have heart disease know very little about the lethal role of emotional stress in both causing and worsening this disease. The popular notion that hard-driving, aggressive people who live life in the fast lane (exhibiting so-called type A behavior) are most vulnerable to heart disease is an oversimplification of a complex problem. Although type A behavior contributes greatly to coronary disease, other emotional factors are equally important.

*Statistics from the *American Heart Association Bulletin.*

In explaining how your emotions affect your heart, this book goes far beyond conventional type A descriptions. It discusses precisely how certain emotional land mines cause stress reactions that can be lethal. We will show how the Sisyphus syndrome, emotional entrapment, and type A behavior can wreck your life and damage your heart. Once you recognize these lifelong traps, you can avoid or minimize them. You may then turn the emotional energy which has been killing you into a positive and vital force for living.

This book is a complete guide for dealing with all the physical and emotional dimensions of the major forms of heart disease: hypertension, angina pectoris, heart attack, and sudden cardiac death. We discuss these conditions, their causes, their diagnoses, their dangers, and their treatments.

Along with case histories, we present excerpts of patients' recollections and actual accounts of their experiences (and their physical and emotional reactions). We've included frequently asked questions with practical answers to help you successfully deal with heart disease.

Then we present our Heartplan—a complete strategy for dealing with heart disease that derails potentially lethal emotions and allows your mind to work for you. This book provides practical advice you can use every day of your life. And it tells you how you might *prevent* heart disease.

Because we rarely see a patient who is physically disabled by heart disease, we tell you how to avoid the tragedy of emotional invalidism and to live a full life even if you have heart disease or have had a heart attack. You can enjoy healthful foods at home and in restaurants, have a full sex life, exercise sensibly; and cope with your work, your family, your friends—and your entire life.

The book has three sections: Part 1 describes The Problem, namely, how heart disease is caused and worsened. Part 2 presents Heartplan. Part 3, Anything Else You Need to Know, discusses surgery, the latest medical advances, your sex life, and the future and includes a chapter for your partner.

Heart disease is a personal and family crisis that often calls forth previously untapped emotional resources. We believe this book can turn your life around. Even if you have not been diagnosed as having heart disease, the ongoing effects of daily stresses, large and small, probably compromise your enjoyment of life. This book will help you use the powers of your mind and body to deal with stress and conquer heart disease to realize your full potential for living. *Heartplan* can help you turn a crisis into a lesson for leading a richer and more satisfying life.

Mark Rubinstein, M.D.
David L. Copen, M.D

Note to the Reader

The diagnosis of heart disease may mean that a family must change its life-style, how family members deal with stresses, and how they live and deal with each other. Heart disease often affects an entire family, and everything in these pages is written for both patient and family. Reading *Heartplan* together can spark ideas and helpful discussions you never thought possible.

PART 1
The Problem

1

The Heart-Mind Connection

That a psychiatrist and cardiologist would write this book is the most natural thing in the world. After all, the heart and mind are intimately linked. For example, consider the following incidents.

> A 72-year-old man brought his wife into the emergency room. Breathing heavily, she was in great distress, and her condition was obviously serious. She quickly worsened and died within an hour. The moment the intern told the man that his wife was dead, the husband's eyes bulged, he turned pallid and sweaty and then collapsed. The staff tried to revive him, but the man's pulse grew weaker. An electrocardiogram (ECG) showed marked abnormalities indicating severe, sudden heart damage. An hour later, the man's heart was quivering uselessly, and, despite all efforts to resuscitate him, he died.

The British Medical Journal (1969) reported the following scientific study:

> The ECGs of some healthy people were continuously monitored as they drove their cars in routine traffic. The tracings showed

the onset of erratic rhythms and other cardiac abnormalities usually seen in people with longstanding heart disease. These abnormalities were also noted in normal people monitored while subjected to the stress of public speaking.

The final illustration of the heart-mind connection is an actual case history:

Steve Bauer* came for a consultation because he had experienced chest pains for nearly a year. Various tests, including angiography, revealed major obstruction in three coronary arteries. Steve was informed of his range of treatment options and decided against bypass surgery. He chose to make our Heartplan a way of life so that he could deal with his advanced heart disease.

Over the next year Steve lost 52 pounds and began jogging. Although he reached the point of completing the course of the New York City marathon, during the race he developed pressing chest pains which persisted for hours. The next morning an EKG revealed that he had suffered a heart attack.

Unshaken by this news, Steve left the office, determined to defy his disease and live by Heartplan. He continued with the conventional aspects of the plan (dieting, exercising, and not smoking) but also decided to concentrate more fully on certain emotional aspects of his life. Steve identified the stresses in his daily life and developed ways to handle them. Five years later, he is still running marathons, and he enjoys a full life.

These three vignettes illustrate how the heart and mind are intimately connected. Look at Steve Bauer, for instance. Although we don't recommend a "marathon" approach and certainly feel that Steve used poor judgment in delaying treatment after he experienced chest pains, his experience clearly demonstrates the vital power of the mind over the body. Steve corrected certain conventional life-style mistakes involving diet and exercise and got very much better as a result. But he did more—he also changed crucial mental attitudes. Although he already had a serious heart condition, Steve Bauer was able to defy the odds and his illness.

*All patients' names have been changed.

Throughout history, people have recognized the connections between the heart and mind. The Sumerians viewed the heart as the source of thought, emotions, will—the soul—and the organ from which conscience, determination, and memory (all mental attributes) have their origins. Many ancient civilizations believed that virtue and vice, humility and pride, good and evil, all came from the heart.

Today, we express the unity of the heart and mind in our folklore, songs, and everyday expressions. We talk about heartache, heartbreak, heaviness of the heart, the heart of a lion, to learn by heart, to warm one's heart, to win one's heart, and scores of other phrases.

This book explains these crucial heart-mind connections, detailing how negative emotions influence your heart and help bring about or worsen heart disease. The book will then illustrate how to use the powers of your mind to deal with stressful, negative emotions and convert them into a positive plan for experiencing life to the fullest.

This book is about living life. In a very real way, it's mind over matter.

2

Your Heart in Health and Disease

Before we discuss what can go wrong with your cardiovascular system, we must examine the normal heart and normal blood vessels. The word *cardiovascular* has two parts: *cardio* means heart, and *vascular* means blood vessels.

The heart is a muscle. It functions as a pump to circulate blood throughout the body, but it is a pump like no other on earth. Each day it beats more than a hundred thousand times, going month after month and year after year without resting, and never needing lubrication or maintenance.

An electrical system in the heart controls the rate at which it beats. The normal resting heart rate is between 50 and 75 beats per minute: with exercise, it can go as high as 200 beats per minute, pumping five times as much blood as when you are resting. The heart has four interior valves that keep blood flowing in the proper direction. This nonstop pumping keeps a constant pressure head going through nearly 60,000 miles of blood vessels. Freshly oxygenated blood is pumped out the left side of the heart into the aorta, the largest artery of the body. From there, it passes through a network of smaller blood vessels, reaching every cell throughout the body. Blood delivers nourishment (food and oxygen) to the cells and removes cell waste products. Once depleted of food and oxygen, the blood travels through a series of veins back to the right side of the heart. From there, it is pumped out through the pulmonary artery to the lungs, where it takes on oxygen, returns to the heart, and is again pumped out to the body.

This amazing vascular network depends on the heart to pump blood at a constant pressure, with no back-ups and no failure. Thus the heart must pump at a slow rate when you sleep (when the body's needs are minimal) and at a very quick rate when you jog (when the demand for oxygen and food increases). All this is controlled by the brain, which acts as a field commander, regulating the rate and force of the heart's action to meet the body's requirements.

About Blood Pressure

Blood pressure is the force generated by the heart to pump blood through the blood vessels. Each time the heart muscle contracts, the pressure rises. When the heart relaxes, the pressure falls.

When taking your blood pressure, the doctor or nurse simply measures the pressure when the heart contracts (the *systolic* pressure) and the pressure when the heart completely relaxes (the *diastolic* pressure). You can feel this pressure by taking your pulse with your index and third fingers placed over the radial artery of your wrist. A blood pressure reading of 120/80 is read as 120 "over" 80; 120 is the systolic pressure, and 80 is the diastolic pressure.

About Heart Disease

Heart disease can affect any component of the heart. For example, abnormalities of the electrical system cause abnormal cardiac rhythms called *arrhythmias*. When the valves become diseased, one of two things can happen: the valves may leak, resulting in blood flow in the wrong direction, or the valves may narrow, preventing adequate amounts of blood from passing through to the rest of the body. A diseased heart muscle becomes weak and can no longer pump blood to the vital organs, resulting in congestive heart failure.

The most common heart disease in our society is *coronary artery disease*. Approximately one in four Americans over the age of 60 is affected by it. Almost everything that you read in newspapers and magazines about preventing and treating heart disease concerns coronary artery disease. It is a disease of the blood vessels that supply the heart muscle, and it results from *atherosclerosis*, or hardening of the arteries.

Atherosclerosis

Atherosclerosis is a silent assassin caused by a slow buildup of fatty deposits (plaques) on the inner lining of arterial walls. These deposits, composed mostly of *cholesterol*, accumulate and narrow the blood vessels in which they form. (See Figure 1.)

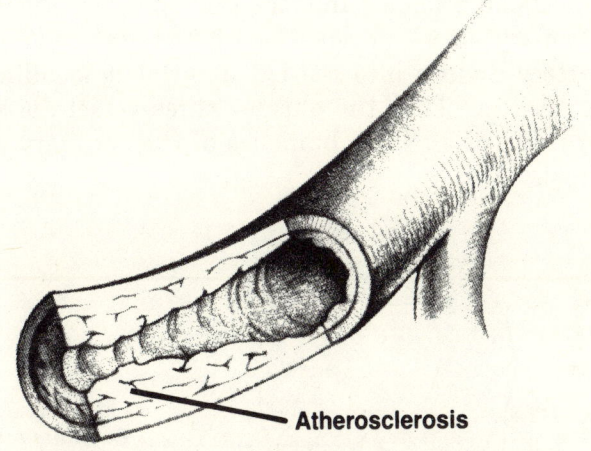

Figure 1.

Atherosclerosis is a slow but steady process that you don't feel happening. Severe narrowing takes many years to develop, although the process begins early. Autopsies on men who died in the Korean War revealed fatty streaks on their inner arterial walls at an average age of 22 years old!

At birth, the inner arterial lining is smooth and open, but small injuries may occur as time passes that result in the steady buildup of plaque on the arteries' inner surfaces. Plaque consists of the repair materials deposited by the body at these minor injuries *plus* cholesterol, a fatty material that circulates in the blood. Plaque reduces the flexibility of the arteries and, once formed, hastens the further accumulation of fatty material. The process may be compared to rust or lime collecting in a pipe, which explains the use of the common phrase "hardening of the arteries." The slow but steady laying down of artery-narrowing plaque is accelerated by too much cholesterol in your diet, by high blood pressure, by cigarette smoking, and by certain chemicals released into your bloodstream when you are under stress.

Why the Heart Is Vulnerable

The heart, like every other part of the body, requires blood and oxygen. Unfortunately, the blood contained within its chambers does not feed the heart tissue itself. Rather, the coronary arteries, blood vessels branching off the aorta, course over the heart's surface, sending small branches into the heart muscle. Figure 2 shows the two coronary arteries branching off the aorta. The left main coronary artery divides into the left anterior descending and left circumflex arteries. Thus the phrase "three-vessel disease" refers to the narrowing of all three branches of the coronary arteries by atherosclerosis.

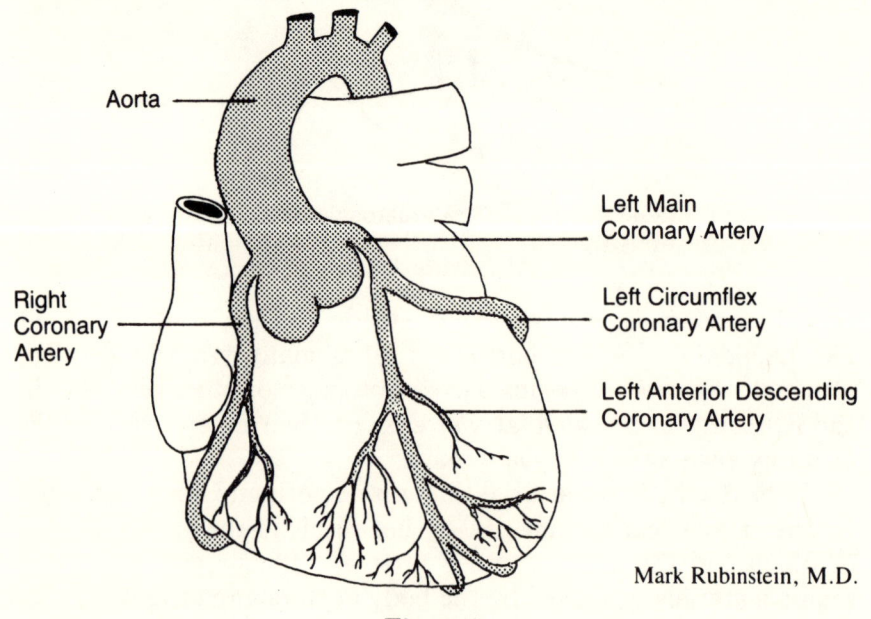

Mark Rubinstein, M.D.

Figure 2.

When the coronary arteries become severely narrowed by atherosclerotic buildup, symptoms such as chest pain may develop. A blood clot (a *thrombus*) may suddenly occlude (block) a vessel, causing a heart attack or lethal rhythm disturbance.

Angina versus a Heart Attack

Angina is chest pain that generally warns that the heart muscle is not getting enough oxygen. A *heart attack* occurs when no oxygen gets to part of the heart muscle (due to total blockage of a coronary artery) and that part of the heart muscle dies and turns to scar tissue.

Angina

Angina pectoris occurs when a coronary artery becomes severely narrowed. The heart receives enough oxygen when you rest but not when you are exerting or are emotionally stimulated. Thus chest pains during activity, such as walking or shoveling snow, or emotional excitement, result. The heart is demanding more oxygen, and the pain subsides shortly after the exertion or excitement stops. Usually angina pectoris develops when a coronary artery is one-third of its normal size. An angina "attack" usually involves a dull, pressing pain beneath the breast bone, described by some patients as "burning" or "squeezing." The pain may radiate to your left arm or jaw, and it may be felt on the left side of your chest. The pain usually, but not always, begins during activity or when you are emotionally upset. Some angina pains may occur at rest, often indicating severe narrowing of the coronary arteries and preceding a full-blown heart attack.

Angina pain is usually alleviated by rest. Pain persisting longer than a few minutes may herald the onset of a heart attack. If you experience such pain, you should go to a hospital emergency room for a complete medical examination, since a prolonged episode of pain may mean you are having a heart attack.

Heart Attack

A heart attack occurs when the flow of blood to the heart is completely blocked. Much more than chest pain occurs; the heart muscle itself is damaged, and part of it is destroyed. A heart attack is technically called a *myocardial infarction* (MI). (*Myo* means muscle; *cardio* means heart; *infarction* means death of the tissue.)

Blockage of the coronary arteries can occur in several ways. A gradual deposit of plaque over years may narrow an artery so that it becomes completely blocked. Or a blood clot may form in an already narrowed artery and block the flow of blood to the part of the heart muscle supplied by that artery. Or the flow may be blocked by a sudden spasm of the coronary artery.

As Figure 3 shows, a severely narrowed coronary artery can lead to angina pectoris, and, if the artery is occluded, a heart attack may occur. Chapter 6 discusses heart attack onset and symptoms.

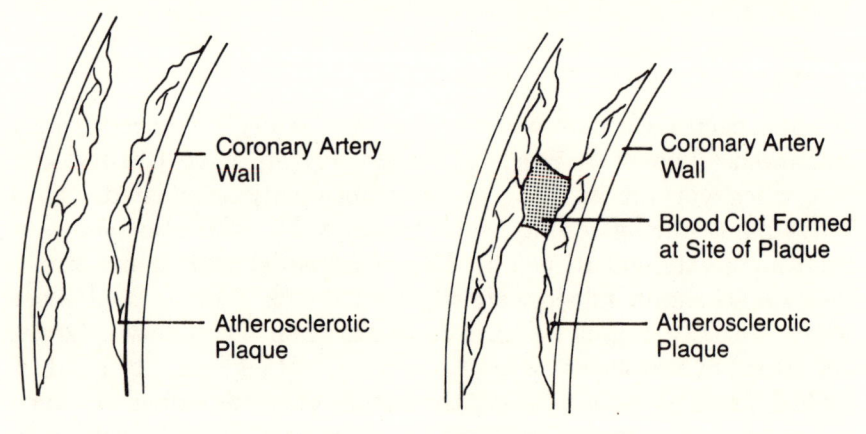

Narrowed coronary artery which may lead to angina pectoris

Blocked coronary artery which can lead to a heart attack (myocardial infarction)

Figure 3.

Diagnosing Cardiovascular Disease

Because atherosclerosis usually develops slowly, without dramatic symptoms, diagnosis is difficult in its early stages. Sometimes, the first symptoms are a heart attack or stroke, by which time irreversible destruction of tissue has occurred and death may be the final outcome.

Fortunately, in many cases of coronary artery narrowing, the telltale symptoms of angina pectoris occur, allowing for diagnosis and appropriate treatment. Today's sophisticated diagnostic techniques allow discovery of many cases of cardiovascular disease even before symptoms occur. The following are the major tests used to diagnose coronary heart disease.

Electrocardiography

The electrocardiogram (ECG)—a recording of the electrical activity of the heart—is a test familiar to most people. Usually done in a doctor's office, it should be part of any routine physical examination, whether or not you have cardiac symptoms. The tracings obtained can sometimes suggest a number of abnormalities, including a previous heart attack, enlargement of the heart, or an inadequate blood supply to the heart muscle because of coronary artery narrowing.

Exercise Stress Test

An exercise stress test uses the ECG recorded during exercise. Your ECG tracing may be normal while you are at rest but show signs of insufficient coronary blood flow during exertion, when your heart requires additional oxygen. The test uses continuous monitoring of the ECG during exercise on a treadmill or bicycling machine. This test can pick up abnormalities when the coronary artery is narrowed to less than half its normal width.

Many physicians think that the exercise stress test is not a necessary part of a routine physical examination. They recommend it only if you have recurrent chest pain or if many coronary risk factors make you a probable candidate for significant narrowing of the coronary arteries. The test is often recommended before beginning a vigorous exercise program (jogging, rowing, swimming). It is also recommended if you are over 40 years old and lead a sedentary life, if you have a family history of angina pectoris or heart attacks, if you smoke cigarettes or have diabetes.

Nuclear Cardiac Scans

Nuclear cardiac scans use small amounts of radioactive isotopes to evaluate the blood supply and function of the heart.

The *thallium scan* measures blood flow to the heart muscle both at rest and during exercise. The patient exercises on a treadmill. At the point of maximal exertion, a small amount of radioactive thallium 201 is injected intravenously. This material is quickly taken up by the heart muscle and stays there until it is excreted by the body. A special scintillation camera detects the gamma rays emitted by the thallium isotope, and a computer translates the information into pictures. If the blood vessel supplying a certain area of heart muscle is narrowed, the concentration of thallium in that area will be low. The test gives an accurate picture of the blood flow to various segments of heart muscle.

A *MUGA* (multiple gated acquisition) *scan* evaluates heart muscle function. A substance that stays in the blood, technicium, is injected intravenously. A special camera visualizes this substance in the chambers of the heart and produces a picture of the heart contracting. Any part of the heart muscle that has an inadequate blood supply will be seen contracting improperly. When performed at rest, this test gives a good idea of how much heart muscle has been damaged by heart attacks.

Thallium and MUGA scans increase the accuracy of an exercise stress test and can pick up very slight degrees of insufficient blood supply to the heart.

Coronary Angiography

Coronary angiography uses high-resolution X-ray equipment to obtain crystal clear pictures of the coronary arteries. A catheter (a long plastic tube about as wide as a straw) is inserted into the bloodstream via an arm or groin artery and threaded through the blood vessels to reach the heart. Opaque dye is then injected directly into the coronary arteries and X-ray motion pictures are taken. This is the only way to define precisely the anatomy of the coronary arteries; coronary angiography provides a clear picture of the severity of coronary artery obstruction.

Echocardiogram

Another important test is the echocardiogram. This test bounces high-frequency sound waves off the heart (in the same way that surface ships search for submarines with sonar). A picture is then constructed of the reflected waves, giving an accurate image of the cardiac chambers and valves. Echocardiograms are the best method to detect abnormal valve function. They also give a good estimate of muscle damage from a heart attack. Recent advances in echocardiography now allow cardiologists to detect narrowed or leaking heart valves.

When heart disease involves a disturbance of the electrical system of the heart, the heart's rhythm can be accurately evaluated using the two following methods.

Holter Monitor

This consists of a lightweight, portable tape recorder that can be worn beneath the clothing. It records every heartbeat for hours; the information is then processed by a computer and analyzed by a cardiologist. This test is used to detect the cause of symptoms such as palpitations and to evaluate a patient's response to drug therapy.

Trans-Telephonic Monitoring

Some patients experience sudden bursts of cardiac irregularities and palpitations. The second method for evaluating heart rhythm is trans-telephonic monitoring (TTM); TTM allows patients to record their heart rhythms when they are experiencing symptoms. The device is the size of a pack of cigarettes and is worn with two electrodes attached to the patient's chest. When a patient experiences symptoms (dizziness, palpitations, or faintness), she or he can activate the device and record the heart's rhythm. The patient then telephones a central number and plays the unit into a recorder so that doctors can accurately diagnose the arrhythmia.

Risk Evaluation

Physicians are increasingly optimistic that these innovative techniques can accurately pinpoint diseased coronary arteries and hearts and can decipher any irregularities of rhythm. But since hypertension, atherosclerosis, and the beginnings of heart disease are often deceptively silent, many people have no idea that potentially deadly processes are taking place within their bodies. Thus it is crucial to know as much as you can about your risks and how to deal with them—whether or not you have any symptoms.

3
The Risks: How They Affect You

Over the years, physicians have learned that some people have a high risk of developing heart disease. Risk factors are really the sum profile of your day-to-day living habits, along with certain facts about your medical condition and history.

Risks You Can't Do Anything about

Certain risk factors are simply beyond your control, although knowing about them is important. Awareness of the risks can motivate you to modify other risk factors that you *can* control. The following are the risk factors beyond your control.

Age
The chance of developing heart disease increases as you get older. Atherosclerosis and the factors contributing to its formation take their toll as the years go by, although it is a mistake to think that only very old people suffer from heart disease. Nearly a quarter of the victims of fatal heart attacks are below age 65, and many are under 40.

Gender

Coronary heart disease is more common in men than in women, although after women pass through menopause, the difference is less pronounced. In the past several years, the incidence of cardiovascular disease in women has increased. Many physicians believe that certain social trends are instrumental in this emerging pattern; for example, more women than ever before are smoking—particularly younger women—and more women now work at high-stress jobs.

Your Family and Heredity

Heart disease runs in families. A history of sudden deaths or of illnesses such as high blood pressure, heart attacks, and strokes is indeed a risk factor. But if your parents and grandparents lived well into their eighties and then died of other causes, your chances of developing heart disease are slight.

Current Heart Disease

If you have already been diagnosed as having angina pectoris, severe coronary atherosclerosis, and hypertension, then you are at high risk for cardiovascular disease. Although you can't "undo" your own medical history, you *can* do a great deal about the modifiable risk factors, as we shall demonstrate in Part II.

Diabetes

Diabetes, a disease in which the body does not make proper use of carbohydrates (starches and sugars), is caused by a failure of the pancreas to produce enough insulin. Diabetes greatly increases the risk of heart attack and stroke, both because the disease directly affects the cardiovascular system and because it may be associated with a high level of fats in the blood.

Diabetes also hastens the process of hardening of the arteries, although no one knows exactly how. Although there is no way to prevent the onset of diabetes, its effects on the cardiovascular system can be minimized. Controlling diabetes involves adhering to the proper diet, taking prescribed insulin, staying thin, keeping active, and, above all, getting regular medical checkups. Diabetics can do a great deal about diabetes!

Risks You Can Control

Hypertension

Nearly 35 million Americans have consistently elevated blood pressure—hypertension. This condition, often called "the silent killer," rarely has characteristic symptoms, so most people don't know that they have high blood pressure. The diagnosis requires nothing more complicated than multiple blood pressure readings by your physician or by a nurse.

Normal blood pressure is usually below 150/90, although the reading varies depending on certain conditions such as your age and the circumstances under which your blood pressure is taken. For instance, a reading in a supermarket, where there is noise and a great deal of activity, will probably differ from a reading taken while you are resting quietly in your doctor's examining room—although anxiety can make some people's blood pressure skyrocket when they enter a doctor's office. Most physicians agree that persistently elevated blood pressure measurements are needed to establish the diagnosis of hypertension.

The cardiovascular system of a hypertensive person is damaged by high blood pressure. Blood vessels constrict and eventually become thickened and hardened. The heart must work harder to pump blood through these vessels, and the heart muscle thickens, eventually weakening. After twenty or thirty years of high blood pressure, heart failure may occur because the heart has been damaged by chronic overwork. Untreated hypertension makes you four times more prone to severe atherosclerosis, which can eventually lead to angina pectoris or a heart attack.

Hypertension often runs in families. This inborn tendency may be triggered by other factors such as prolonged stress, obesity, excess salt consumption, and a sedentary life-style. Job-related stress is an important contributor to elevated blood pressure. A well-known Boston University Medical Center study found that air-traffic controllers had four times as much hypertension as did the public at large.

Table salt—or any food containing a great deal of sodium—may contribute to high blood pressure. (Some controversy about this has recently surfaced.) Sodium may cause the body to retain water, thus increasing the "vascular load" that the heart must pump, causing more work for an already overworked heart.

Although hypertension is a major risk factor for the development of heart disease and strokes, it can be controlled. Losing weight, restricting salt intake, and regular exercise often lower blood pressure and can make a great difference for many patients. People with more resistant cases can be successfully treated with medication.

Cholesterol

The level of cholesterol and other fats in the blood is one of the most important risk indicators for cardiovascular disease. As mentioned earlier, atherosclerotic plaques are partly composed of cholesterol, which is deposited in the walls of coronary arteries, causing narrowing and stiffening. The narrowed vessels are largely responsible for preventing blood from getting through to the heart tissue.

The presence of cholesterol in your body is not harmful. In fact, it is a normal part of blood and body tissues; it is the material from which sex hormones are derived. Although you get most of your cholesterol from the foods you eat, your liver produces some cholesterol, even if you have absolutely no cholesterol in your diet. (Triglycerides are another group of fatty substances that probably play a minor role in promoting cardiovascular disease.) Too much of these fatty substances in your bloodstream can promote clogging of your arteries, thereby increasing your risk of having a heart attack.

Most Americans have too much cholesterol in their bloodstreams. But how much is too much? According to the U.S. Department of Health, Education and Welfare, the normal level for Americans is between 180 and 230 milligrams per 100 cubic milliliters of blood. But this is normal for a population where one out of four people over age 60 has heart disease! Today, physicians recommend keeping your blood cholesterol below 200 milligrams. Many studies have shown that the lower your cholesterol level, the less likely you are to develop heart disease.

Simply measuring cholesterol may not be enough. To be transported in your blood, cholesterol must be bound to a protein; these fat-protein complexes are called *lipoproteins*. One such transporter, high-density lipoprotein (HDL), may be crucial in assessing coronary risk. HDL seems to protect the body against coronary artery disease by carrying cholesterol away from blood vessel walls and sending it to the liver for excretion. Thus doctors don't simply assess the amount of cholesterol in your bloodstream; they also measure the amount of HDL as compared to the total cholesterol. People with high levels of HDL and low total cholesterol have the lowest risk of having heart attacks. HDL levels are higher than normal in long-distance runners and in women, and both of these groups have low risk for heart attacks. HDL is increased by vigorous exercise and, possibly, by small amounts of alcohol—but not too much!

Scientists are now searching for a way to raise the level of HDL in your blood. At the present, short of becoming a long-distance runner, there is no sure way to create a more favorable balance.

The American Heart Association recommends that you limit the quantity of cholesterol and saturated fats in your diet to reduce your blood cholesterol. Eat no more than three egg yolks a week, use low fat or skim milk instead of whole milk, and limit your meat intake to no more than 6 ounces of veal, poultry or fish each day. We will discuss diet and your heart at greater length in Step 6 of our Heartplan.

Smoking

Cigarette smoking is one of the most important—and controllable—risk factors for developing heart disease, especially in younger people, ages 35 to 50. It is *the most critical* heart attack risk factor that can be totally eliminated.

Precisely how cigarettes damage the heart is not completely known. Carbon monoxide produced by the cigarette is taken into the bloodstream and can easily interfere with oxygen delivery to the cells. When you smoke, your blood is deprived of oxygen: if your heart is already oxygen-deprived because of coronary artery narrowing, you're treading on dangerous ground. Nicotine, which is inhaled by all smokers, constricts the blood vessels, raising blood pressure and making the heart work more vigorously as it pumps oxygen-deprived blood through the system. Smoking can also increase your pulse rate and cause premature heartbeats as well as irregular rhythms of the heart.

If you smoke more than a pack of cigarettes a day, you increase your risk of heart disease threefold. If you survive a heart attack but continue to smoke cigarettes, you double your chances of having a second heart attack. If you are a young man or woman who smokes, you double your risk for heart disease. The surgeon general's report states that a young woman who both smokes and uses oral contraceptives multiplies her risk by a factor of 10. This risk increases even more with age, so that a woman over 40 who smokes and takes birth control pills treads on very thin ice.

Although we don't yet know precisely how cigarette smoking shortens life, quitting smoking has very beneficial effects. If you give up cigarettes, you have an almost immediate drop in your mortality rate from heart attacks. After ten years off cigarettes, your risk of dying from heart disease approaches that of a non-smoker. Giving up cigarettes at *any* age pays enormous dividends, improving your health and your life expectancy.

Obesity and a Sedentary Life-Style

Being overweight is often associated with having increased amounts of cholesterol and high blood pressure. These risk factors are usually found in combination, and they increase your risk for developing heart disease.

Although not a direct risk factor, lack of regular exercise is often associated with being overweight, which in turn often goes hand in hand with hypertension and high levels of blood cholesterol and triglycerides. Epidemiologic studies have shown that people who engage in strenuous activity a few times each week have a low incidence of heart disease and sudden death.

The Pill

Oral contraceptives (OCs), or "the pill," have been associated with an increased risk of heart attack in women over 40. Oral contraceptives promote the retention of salt which in turn raises blood pressure and may enhance blood-clot formation. The pill is also known to raise triglyceride levels while decreasing the levels of HDL. If you are a woman approaching age 40 and using oral contraceptives, consider your other risk factors and then, in consultation with your doctor, decide if your situation warrants changing to another form of birth control.

About These Risk Factors

No one knows the precise ways in which all these risk factors contribute to any person's developing heart disease, nor is it exactly known how they may operate in combination with each other.

Remember that these risk factors are statistics for large groups of people. When applied to any individual, they may be less valid indicators of risk. Since the list is a long one, anyone will fit into at least one or more of these high-risk categories. Being in a high-risk group does not mean you will develop the disease, it is simply a statistical indication of possible risk for developing symptoms.

Just as not everyone in the high-risk groups develops heart disease, no risk factors in your profile is no guarantee of immunity. There is no sure way right now to tell who will develop heart disease. Every person may be a potential victim. We recently treated a 54-year-old executive who seemed to have no risk factors. He never smoked, ate little cholesterol, had normal blood pressure, and exercised regularly. Yet he had a major heart attack, and two of the coronary arteries supplying his heart were severely diseased. Closer examination revealed one risk factor: a high-stress occupation to which he responded with extreme determination, competitiveness, and workaholic patterns.

Cardiovascular disease is the result of a highly complicated mosaic of risk factors interacting with each other. The emotions are one of the most important factors.

> Peter Fitzpatrick, a 50-year-old sales executive with a large corporation, awoke late on a Monday morning and hurried through his early routines. He'd dreaded this day for months—he was to present a report of his division's sales over the preceding year, and volume had been on the downturn for 18 months.
>
> Moving briskly toward the platform after parking his car, he broke into a trot because the passengers were already boarding the train. Covering the last 30 yards in record time, he hustled his way on board moments before the train pulled away. Once seated, he noticed a sense of tightness in his chest, but thought nothing of it, since he was out of breath and huffing mightily. Within a minute, the feeling subsided.

Later that afternoon, as he was presenting his report at the conference, the sensation returned. Peter took an antacid tablet, thinking he'd developed indigestion because he'd rushed his lunch in the short break between the morning and afternoon sessions. Peter was so tense and involved in the conference that he barely heeded the uncomfortable but tolerable feeling.

Over the next few days the tightness returned each time Peter exerted himself or became emotionally upset. He felt it when climbing the stairs from his basement to the kitchen and again when he was scurrying from his office to Grand Central Station to catch the 5:30 train to his suburban Connecticut home. It became especially severe, producing a feeling of someone pressing on his chest, when the executive vice-president of his division criticized Peter's report during a miniconference held after the sales meeting.

Over the next few days the pain became more frequent and pressing, prompting Peter to visit his physician. An examination revealed very little, but his doctor suggested that Peter have certain tests. A treadmill stress test showed some minor changes in his ECG, and coronary angiography revealed significant narrowing of two coronary arteries. The diagnosis was confirmed: Peter had angina pectoris.

Let's look at Peter's risk profile to see where he fits into the picture for developing heart disease. As a 50-year-old white male, Peter was at a higher risk than the general population. More important, Peter's father, now in his seventies and doing well, had suffered a mild heart attack while in his late fifties. Peter's family history put him in the high-risk category.

Peter had been in good health up to that point. He had no history of diabetes or hypertension, although he was certain his blood pressure shot to the ceiling each time he went to the office.

Peter's cholesterol level was a revealing 260—higher than that recommended by the American Heart Association, but not that much higher than the level of many affluent Americans who eat plenty of red meat and dairy products. More important, Peter had a high ratio of cholesterol to HDL. This put him into a higher-risk category than his cholesterol reading alone would indicate.

Peter smoked a pack of cigarettes each day for twenty-five years, but he'd stopped smoking two years earlier. This combination placed him in a high-risk group, although his chances of developing heart disease would have been greater had he not quit.

Peter was not severely overweight, but he was about 15 to 20 pounds too heavy for a man of his height and frame. He felt that a significant part of his weight gain had taken place during the two years since he'd quit smoking. (His wife disagreed, saying he'd been overweight for about 10 years.)

Peter had last exercised regularly five years earlier, when he'd begun a program of jogging. He stopped after six months because of an inflamed knee and hadn't replaced the jogging with any equivalent exercise.

Peter's situation is not out of step with that of many American men of his age and social standing. His risk profile combined moderate and high-risk factors, some of which he dealt with, others of which he ignored.

We couldn't say that Peter's life-style, eating habits, or physical condition were outstandingly bad or that this combination of factors placed him at inordinate risk. Literally millions of people have similar risk profiles. Yet on that May morning prior to his sales conference, Peter's heart began to cry out. His body began signaling that it could take no more. Peter had developed heart disease.

We've focused on one crucial element in the composite of factors that led to Peter Fitzpatrick's disease—ongoing *emotional stress* in his daily life: Peter felt that his work was the bane of his existence. It was demanding and dreary, providing neither satisfaction nor sense of accomplishment. Though he earned a fine living, Peter Fitzpatrick considered his job a dead-end position offering only tension, frustration, and the realization that he'd gone as far as he could go. Despite working sixty hours each week, Peter would never be promoted—and he knew it was too late to change his life's course.

Before discussing the vital issue of your emotions, we will present RISKO, a heart-hazard appraisal developed by the American Heart Association—see pages 24-26. RISKO is based on the Framingham, Stanford, and Chicago heart disease studies, three

MEN

Find the column for your age group. Everyone starts with a score of 10 points. Work down the page *adding* points to your score or *subtracting* points from your score.

	54 OR YOUNGER	55 OR OLDER
	STARTING SCORE 10	STARTING SCORE 10

1. WEIGHT

Locate your weight category in the table below. If you are in . . .

- weight category A
- weight category B
- weight category C
- weight category D

	54 OR YOUNGER	55 OR OLDER
	SUBTRACT 2	SUBTRACT 2
	SUBTRACT 1	ADD 0
	ADD 1	ADD 1
	ADD 2	ADD 3
	EQUALS ☐	EQUALS ☐

2. SYSTOLIC BLOOD PRESSURE

Use the "first" or "higher" number from your most recent blood pressure measurement. If you do not know your blood pressure, estimate it by using the letter for your weight category. If your blood pressure is . . .

- A 119 or less
- between 120 and 139
- between 140 and 159
- D 160 or greater

	SUBTRACT 1	SUBTRACT 5
	ADD 0	SUBTRACT 2
	ADD 0	ADD 1
	ADD 1	ADD 4
	EQUALS ☐	EQUALS ☐

3. BLOOD CHOLESTEROL LEVEL

Use the number from your most recent blood cholesterol test. If you do not know your blood cholesterol, estimate it by using the letter for your weight category. If your blood cholesterol is . . .

- A 199 or less
- between 200 and 224
- between 225 and 249
- D 250 or higher

	SUBTRACT 2	SUBTRACT 1
	SUBTRACT 1	SUBTRACT 1
	ADD 0	ADD 0
	ADD 1	ADD 0
	EQUALS ☐	EQUALS ☐

4. CIGARETTE SMOKING

If you . . .

(If you smoke a pipe, but not cigarettes, use the same score adjustment as those cigarette smokers who smoke less than a pack a day.)

- do not smoke
- smoke less than a pack a day
- smoke a pack a day
- smoke more than a pack a day

	SUBTRACT 1	SUBTRACT 2
	ADD 0	SUBTRACT 1
	ADD 1	ADD 0
	ADD 2	ADD 3
	FINAL SCORE EQUALS ☐	FINAL SCORE EQUALS ☐

WEIGHT TABLE FOR MEN

Look for your height (without shoes) in the far left column and then read across to find the category into which your weight (in indoor clothing) would fall.

YOUR HEIGHT FT IN	WEIGHT CATEGORY (lbs.)			
	A	B	C	D
5 1	up to 123	124-148	149-173	174 plus
5 2	up to 126	127-152	153-178	179 plus
5 3	up to 129	130-156	157-182	183 plus
5 4	up to 132	133-160	161-186	187 plus
5 5	up to 135	136-163	164-190	191 plus
5 6	up to 139	140-168	169-196	197 plus
5 7	up to 144	145-174	175-203	204 plus
5 8	up to 148	149-179	180-209	210 plus
5 9	up to 152	153-184	185-214	215 plus
5 10	up to 157	158-190	191-221	222 plus
5 11	up to 161	162-194	195-227	228 plus
6 0	up to 165	166-199	200-232	233 plus
6 1	up to 170	171-205	206-239	240 plus
6 2	up to 175	176-211	212-246	247 plus
6 3	up to 180	181-217	218-253	254 plus
6 4	up to 185	186-223	224-260	261 plus
6 5	up to 190	191-229	230-267	268 plus
6 6	up to 195	196-235	236-274	275 plus
ESTIMATE OF SYSTOLIC BLOOD PRESSURE	119 or less	120 to 139		160 or more
ESTIMATE OF BLOOD CHOLESTEROL	199 or less	200 to 224		250 or more

Because both blood pressure and blood cholesterol are related to weight, an estimate of these risk factors for each weight category is printed at the bottom of the table.

THE RISKS: HOW THEY AFFECT YOU

WOMEN

Find the column for your age group. Everyone starts with a score of 10 points. Work down the page *adding* points to your score or *subtracting* points from your score.

	54 OR YOUNGER	55 OR OLDER
	STARTING SCORE [10]	STARTING SCORE [10]

1. WEIGHT

Locate your weight category in the table below. If you are in . . .

weight category A	SUBTRACT 2	SUBTRACT 2
weight category B	SUBTRACT 1	SUBTRACT 1
weight category C	ADD 1	ADD 0
weight category D	ADD 2	ADD 1
	EQUALS ☐	EQUALS ☐

2. SYSTOLIC BLOOD PRESSURE

Use the "first" or "higher" number from your most recent blood pressure measurement. If you do not know your blood pressure, estimate it by using the letter for your weight category. If your blood pressure is . . .

A — 119 or less	SUBTRACT 2	SUBTRACT 3
between 120 and 139	SUBTRACT 1	ADD 0
between 140 and 159	ADD 0	ADD 3
D — 160 or greater	ADD 1	ADD 6
	EQUALS ☐	EQUALS ☐

3. BLOOD CHOLESTEROL LEVEL

Use the number from your most recent blood cholesterol test. If you do not know your blood cholesterol, estimate it by using the letter for your weight category. If your blood cholesterol is . . .

A — 199 or less	SUBTRACT 1	SUBTRACT 3
between 200 and 224	ADD 0	SUBTRACT 1
between 225 and 249	ADD 0	ADD 1
D — 250 or higher	ADD 1	ADD 3
	EQUALS ☐	EQUALS ☐

4. CIGARETTE SMOKING

If you . . .

do not smoke	SUBTRACT 1	SUBTRACT 2
smoke less than a pack a day	ADD 0	SUBTRACT 1
smoke a pack a day	ADD 1	ADD 1
smoke more than a pack a day	ADD 2	ADD 4
	EQUALS ☐	EQUALS ☐

5. ESTROGEN USE

Birth control pills and hormone drugs contain estrogen. A few examples are: *Premarin *Ogan *Menstranol *Provera *Evex *Menest *Estinyl *Meurium

- Have you ever taken estrogen for five or more years in a row?
- Are you age 35 years or older and are now taking estrogen?

No to both questions	ADD 0	ADD 0
Yes to one or both questions	ADD 1	ADD 3

	FINAL SCORE EQUALS ☐	FINAL SCORE EQUALS ☐

WEIGHT TABLE FOR WOMEN

Look for your height (without shoes) in the far left column and then read across to find the category into which your weight (in indoor clothing) would fall.

YOUR HEIGHT FT IN	WEIGHT CATEGORY (lbs.)			
	A	B	C	D
4 8	up to 101	102-122	123-143	144 plus
4 9	up to 103	104-125	126-146	147 plus
4 10	up to 106	107-128	129-150	151 plus
4 11	up to 109	110-132	133-154	155 plus
5 0	up to 112	113-136	137-158	159 plus
5 1	up to 115	116-139	140-162	163 plus
5 2	up to 119	120-144	145-168	169 plus
5 3	up to 122	123-148	149-172	173 plus
5 4	up to 127	128-154	155-179	180 plus
5 5	up to 131	132-158	159-185	186 plus
5 6	up to 135	136-163	164-190	191 plus
5 7	up to 139	140-168	169-196	197 plus
5 8	up to 143	144-173	174-202	203 plus
5 9	up to 147	148-178	179-207	208 plus
5 10	up to 151	152-182	183-213	214 plus
5 11	up to 155	156-187	188-218	219 plus
6 0	up to 159	160-191	192-224	225 plus
6 1	up to 163	164-196	197-229	230 plus
ESTIMATE OF SYSTOLIC BLOOD PRESSURE	119 or less	120 to 159		160 or more
ESTIMATE OF BLOOD CHOLESTEROL	199 or less	200 to 224		250 or more

Because both blood pressure and blood cholesterol are related to weight, an estimate of these risk factors for each weight category is printed at the bottom of the table.

WHAT YOUR SCORE MEANS

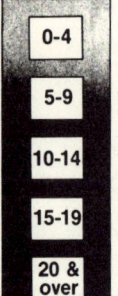

0-4 You have one of the lowest risks of Heart Disease for your age and sex.

5-9 You have a low to moderate risk of Heart Disease for your age and sex but there is some room for improvement.

10-14 You have a moderate to high risk of Heart Disease for your age and sex, with considerable room for improvement on some factors.

15-19 You have a high risk of developing Heart Disease for your age and sex with a great deal of room for improvement on all factors.

20 & over You have a very high risk of developing Heart Disease for your age and sex and should take immediate action on all risk factors.

WARNING
- If you have diabetes, gout or a family history of heart disease, your actual risk will be greater than indicated by this appraisal.
- If you do not know your current blood pressure or blood cholesterol level, you should visit your physician or health center to have them measured. Then figure your score again for a more accurate determination of your risk.
- If you are overweight, have high blood pressure or high blood cholesterol, or smoke cigarettes, your long-term risk of heart disease is increased even if your risk in the next several years is low.

HOW TO REDUCE YOUR RISK

- Try to quit smoking permanently. There are many programs available.
- Have your blood pressure checked regularly, preferably every twelve months after age 40. If your blood pressure is high, see your physician. Remember blood pressure medicine is only effective if taken regularly.
- Consider your daily exercise (or lack of it). A half hour of brisk walking, swimming or other enjoyable activity should not be difficult to fit into your day.
- Give some serious thought to your diet. If you are overweight, or eat a lot of foods high in saturated fat or cholesterol (whole milk, cheese, eggs, butter, fatty foods, fried foods) then changes should be made in your diet. Look for the American Heart Association Cookbook at your local bookstore.
- Visit or write your local Heart Association for further information and copies of free pamphlets on many related subjects including:
  - Reducing your risk of heart attack.
  - Controlling high blood pressure.
  - Eating to keep your heart healthy.
  - How to stop smoking.
  - Exercising for good health.

SOME WORDS OF CAUTION

- If you have diabetes, gout, or a family history of heart disease, your real risk of developing heart disease will be greater than indicated by your RISKO score. If your score is high and you have one or more of these additional problems, you should give particular attention to reducing your risk.
- If you are a woman under 45 years or a man under 35 years of age, your RISKO score represents an upper limit on your real risk of developing heart disease. In this case your real risk is probably lower than indicated by your score.
- If you are a woman whose use of estrogen has contributed to a high RISKO score, you may want to consult your physician. Do not automatically discontinue your prescription.
- Using your weight category to estimate your systolic blood pressure or your blood cholesterol level makes your RISKO score less accurate.
  - Your score will tend to overestimate your risk if your actual values on these two important factors are average for someone of your height and weight.
  - Your score will underestimate your risk if your actual blood pressure or cholesterol level is above average for someone of your height or weight.

long-term research efforts that shed a great deal of light on certain modifiable risk factors for developing heart disease. RISKO is an indicator of risk for adults who do not now show evidence of heart disease.

 The RISKO heart-hazard appraisal is not a substitute for a thorough physical examination and assessment of your situation by your doctor. Rather, you should use it to learn more about your risk of developing heart disease and about ways to reduce this risk. Separate quizzes are given for men and women.

Frequently Asked Questions

We are asked many questions by our patients. Here are some that we are asked almost every day.

I'm a 45-year-old man. My father and grandfather both had heart attacks in their late forties. I'm worried about the chances I too may have heart disease. What should I do?

People with a family history of heart disease have a high risk of developing heart trouble. Thus your history doesn't mean that you will automatically be a heart patient, but it does indicate that you should have a thorough cardiac evaluation and risk-factor assessment. Make a serious effort to reduce your modifiable risk factors such as diet, exercise, smoking, blood pressure, and most important, your susceptibility to stress. Although modifying risk factors provides no guarantees, your long-term outlook is much better if you follow the guidelines set forth in Part II of this book.

I'm a 48-year-old man, and I'm concerned about my blood pressure. Whenever my doctor takes my pressure, it's high. And when I take it on a machine in the supermarket, it's high then too. Yet, at home, it's normal. Which reading should I trust?

Blood pressure is easily affected by emotional tension. Many people become nervous the moment they walk into a physician's office, elevating their blood pressures. Readings may remain high no matter how many times your doctor repeats them. This reading really indicates that when you are under stress, your body reacts as much as, if not more than, your mind.

A quick reading in a supermarket is unlikely to represent your true resting blood pressure. Supermarkets are bright, noisy places with lots of activity, and chances are that you were briskly shopping only moments before recording your blood pressure. This is not an ideal setting. A good setting is where you feel calm, where no loud noises or other stimuli disturb you, and where you are in relaxed circumstances. Such a setting is most likely to be your home.

The readings at home are the most accurate records of your resting blood pressure. The readings in your doctor's office and in the supermarket, however, may be the first real indicators that you are a "hot" reactor to stressful situations.

I'm a 51-year-old man and haven't been able to give up smoking. I'd like to cut down my risk of developing heart disease. Will smoking low-tar cigarettes help?

Probably not. To the best of our knowledge, low-tar cigarettes do *not* reduce the risks for heart disease. A lighted cigarette gives off a host of noxious compounds; some are in gaseous form (hydrogen cyanide, ammonia, and carbon monoxide), and others are particles (such as tar and nicotine). These harmful substances are inhaled by a smoker whether or not the cigarette is low in tar or nicotine. No one really knows what chemical, or combination of chemicals, is responsible for the detrimental effects of cigarette smoking.

By the way, you may be kidding yourself by smoking low-tar cigarettes. To keep your blood concentration of nicotine at its usual level (nicotine is addictive, and, as with any such substance, the blood level must be maintained) you may end up smoking even more low-tar cigarettes than you did regular cigarettes. In the long run you may inhale even more harmful chemicals than you did with regular cigarettes. Let's face it—the best way to protect yourself is to quit smoking.

I'm a 40-year-old woman, and I've been taking birth control pills for quite a few years. There's a lot of heart disease in my family, and I'm concerned. What should I do?

Your concern is understandable. As a woman approaches 40, her risk for heart disease increases if she is using birth control pills. If you are also a smoker, your risk is significantly increased. This warrants a full discussion with your physician. Don't hesitate to express your concern and explore other methods of birth control.

I've heard that drinking coffee increases my risk for heart disease. Is this true?

No. Some early studies indicated that certain men who drank up to seven cups of coffee each day had an increased number of cardiovascular problems. But it turned out that when the results were studied more closely, many of the men who drank that much coffee also smoked more than twice as many cigarettes as non-coffee-drinkers. Cigarettes were the real villain. Heavy coffee drinkers who do not smoke have no higher incidence of heart disease than people who don't drink coffee. Studies released in March 1985 show some correlation between coffee drinking and an increased cholesterol level, but the final results are not in.

I want to cut down on my risk for heart disease. Should I give up drinking?

Giving up alcohol isn't necessary, although heavy drinkers risk liver damage and other long-range effects of overindulgence. For instance, heavy drinking raises your blood triglyceride levels, and, because alcohol has plenty of calories, heavy drinkers run a risk of being overweight, of having elevated triglycerides, and of developing hypertension. All of these may contribute to heart disease.

The good news is that if you drink moderately (2 ounces each day of hard liquor, or its equivalent) you don't increase your risks for cardiovascular disease at all. As a matter of fact, some physicians now point to evidence that moderate drinking may protect you against developing atherosclerosis. The blood levels of high-density lipoproteins (HDLs) seem to be higher in people who drink moderately. The key word is *moderation*: a before-dinner cocktail or a glass or two of wine with dinner may be good for you.

I've heard that aspirin can prevent my having a second heart attack. Is this true?

There is some evidence that small daily doses of aspirin might help to prevent second or third heart attacks. One or two aspirins taken daily may also reduce the risks of having a stroke. Aspirin will prevent anginal pain in some patients and can be helpful in averting "mini-strokes."

I'm 60 years old. Why should I be concerned about lowering my risks at this age?

Controlling your risks at *any* age results in a longer, healthier life. Don't assume that it's too late at age 60. Whatever narrowing has occurred in your arteries can be completely halted, *right now*, if you reduce your risks. There is no reason why you can't live well beyond the traditionally accepted 72 or 74 years.

Coronary heart disease is *not* an inevitable result of getting older. Heart disease is the result of certain *life-style mistakes*, mistakes that can be corrected at any age. Changing them results in a longer and healthier life.

I've heard that heart disease, like many other illnesses, is inherited. If that's true, then why should I worry about lowering my risks?

Perhaps 1 percent of people with heart disease have it as a *direct* result of some genetic problem. Although there can be a family tendency for heart disease, it is not a result of genes only. Rather, a family may be susceptible to developing heart disease, *if* a combination of other factors is present. Those factors are certain excesses such as overeating, too much fat and cholesterol, smoking, hypertension, and, most important, poor stress management.

As for family predispositions, we've observed that life-style excesses (especially overeating and excessive emotional tension) are often passed on from parents to children. These life-style difficulties are crucial in causing or worsening heart disease.

4

Know the Enemy: Stress, the Most Dangerous Risk

We've already established that certain people are prone to the buildup of atherosclerotic plaques in their coronary arteries. Chapter 4 explores how emotional stress may contribute to heart disease.

What Happens When You Are Stressed

When you encounter danger, your brain registers the threat and immediately flashes signals to every part of your body. In an instant, you are prepared for action. This fight-or-flight response to danger is universal; it happens to all people and to every member of the animal kingdom whenever danger threatens. Your mind and body work together for the most basic of all possible purposes: self-preservation.

This fight-or-flight response evokes instant vigilance. You are ready for action. With split-second speed, your body activates a part of your nervous system (the *sympathetic system*) so that you protect yourself by either fighting or fleeing.

A host of physical changes take place during this supercharged moment when your defenses are mobilized. Your pupils dilate, your face flushes, your palms get sweaty, breathing quickens, digestion slows, and blood diverts to your muscles as they swing into a tense, ready-for-action posture.

Along with these changes, the cardiovascular system surges into instant action. Your heart rate increases and your pulse bounds. Your blood pressure soars as more blood is pumped into your tensed muscles and adrenaline pours through your system. Blood tends to clot more easily, and the muscle in the walls of your coronary arteries may spasm, which narrows the vessels.

These spasms, which occur in arteries with or without atherosclerotic narrowing, are believed to be triggered by one of two mechanisms. The brain can signal the nerves that lie within the walls of the coronary arteries to make them constrict. The brain can also command the adrenal glands to pour more adrenaline into this primed system, causing more spasm. These two mechanisms can cause coronary artery constriction, reducing blood flow to the heart. Chest pain (angina pectoris) or, if the blood flow is completely blocked, a heart attack may result.

This partly explains why some heart patients experience angina pains when they become upset. An already-narrowed coronary artery combined with stress-induced spasm can lead to a heart attack and sometimes sudden death. Recall the case of the 72-year-old man who collapsed and died in the emergency room when he was told that his wife had died.

Also, evidence is accumulating that links severe emotional stress with sudden death. Certain laboratory experiments with animals have shown that stimulation of the hypothalamus, part of the brain, can provoke abnormal heart rhythms, even if the animals do not have coronary artery occlusion and their arteries do not spasm. In other words, excess nervous system activity—as can occur in a state of panic—can trigger sudden death, even in someone who does not have atherosclerosis!

You may say, "Okay, you've convinced me that sudden, intense stress is bad for me. It can even kill me. But how often do I run into a situation like that? My stresses are everyday things—an argument with my wife, getting caught in traffic, nothing dramatic." Unfortunately, these everyday things can add up, especially over twenty to thirty years. Also, although we no longer live in caves, our bodies often respond to stresses (even minor ones) in the same primitive ways they have since prehistoric times. For the cave dwellers, this fight-or-flight response had survival value, since they had to be ready for battle or flight as part of their daily experience. Today, this stress-response system is pretty much obsolete; after all, how often do we run into tigers or find our lives truly endangered?

Modern stresses are usually more subtle and prolonged. Our responses are more emotional than physical, and they're usually internalized. We "grin and bear it" and for the most part don't swing into high gear to do battle. For us, getting uptight equals a fight-or-flight response, and many of us are uptight for hours each day. Some people are tense and anxious for weeks at a time—ask any accountant about the four or five weeks before April 15. Some people are nervous and under stress most of the time.

Although our everyday stresses are less dramatic than running into a tiger, we often assume an "attack" posture without even being aware of it. This chronic stress response is something like driving a car in the wrong gear: the wear and tear eventually shows.

The body produces other responses to stress. Adrenaline released by the stress response affects not only the heart. It raises blood pressure and elevates the blood cholesterol level, both of which can hasten atherosclerosis within the coronary arteries. (Studies show that healthy young medical students have sky-high blood cholesterol levels before exams.)

For many people, stress is an ongoing process; for some, it leads to a vicious cycle which contributes to heart disease.

What Is Stress?

Stress is any situation or change in your life that calls for an adaptive response. It can be anything that causes an upset in your emotional and physical equilibrium. As an inevitable part of life, stress cannot be completely avoided.

Often stress is considered negative: a divorce, a death in the family, an early retirement or the loss of a job, the onset of a major illness, or some other unpleasant change in one's circumstances. However, stresses can also be positive: a promotion (which means more responsibility), moving to a new home (adapting to new surroundings, paying the mortgage), having a baby (a major change in one's life), or starting a new business. Most of these positive changes, although stressful, are the exciting spices of life we usually anticipate.

Stress doesn't have to be dramatic. It can be subtle, taking its toll bit by bit, through minor, everyday hassles: excessive noise at home or at work, traffic jams, crowds, long lines at the supermarket or the bank, chronic overwork, an unpleasant colleague at the office, and a variety of trivial hassles and disappointments at home, school, or work.

Not everyone is stressed by the same things. Something that bothers you may be no problem for someone else. As thinking and feeling beings with a uniquely human capacity for abstract ideas and symbols, we can be deeply bothered by intangible yet powerful stressors that have mostly symbolic meanings.

The case of Peter Fitzpatrick, the sales manager discussed in Chapter 3, illustrates how the response to a personal concern can involve a physical stress response, even though Peter's feelings are the main source of his trouble. He demonstrates how potent the mind-body connection can really be.

Peter's work troubles did not concern doing his job. Rather, his problems began three years earlier, when the division vice-president retired. Peter expected to be promoted to that position. Instead, the company recruited a young man from outside the firm. Peter suddenly saw himself locked into a job that no longer offered any real chance for growth. In addition, the newly appointed vice-president was quite critical of Peter, which became a constant source of tension. Peter had trouble coping with his own frustration, his envy of the younger man, and the criticism that seemed mostly unjustified.

In short, Peter's work world suddenly became one of imminent challenge; he was primed for criticism and felt constantly on guard. Peter wasn't afraid that he'd be fired; he was a valuable employee and knew it. Rather, he now encountered enormous pressure to perform in a ten-hour daily span and felt emotionally (and physically) challenged.

"The minute I get to the office I feel myself tense up," Peter said. "I go into a state of total awareness, like a deer being stalked by a lion. I can *feel* my blood pressure rise. My head begins to pound, and I take an aspirin. But that doesn't help.

"Sometimes, at a sales conference, I realize that I'm all tensed up. Every muscle in my body is bunched, like I'm ready to burst. My legs are stiff and my shoulders are hunched. By the end of the day, I *ache* all over from the tension. It's like being on a high wire with no net below me. One slip, and that'll be *it!* I sometimes wonder why it's so terrible to feel I might be criticized? I mean, so what if you make a mistake once in a while? The worst part is that I know the tension comes from inside my head. And there's nothing I can do about it. Why the hell am I so afraid of making a mistake and being criticized? It's getting me sick. It's wearing away at my heart!"

Peter is emotionally vulnerable to criticism; it has some intolerable meaning for him, and he responds to even the threat of criticism with a totally primed fight-or-flight response that has contributed to his developing angina pectoris.

Whether stress is dramatic or a subtle, everyday experience, people handle it either well or badly. Recent research has identified "hot" and "cool" reactors to stressful situations. Some people remain calm in a storm of stress. Others respond heatedly and have unhealthy responses to even the most ordinary stresses. Their minds propel their bodies into prolonged arousal of their stress-response systems, and they develop high blood pressure, racing pulses, tensed muscles, and signs of a "pumped up" nervous system that may even include abnormal heart rhythms.

Major stresses often precede the onset of many serious illnesses. For instance, recently bereaved widows die at a rate nearly 10 times that of women the same age who are unmarried. And most heart attack victims, upon reflection, realize that they have had a major life stress within the preceding two years!

Minor stress can be a culprit too. Recall the experiment in which healthy people's ECGs were monitored while they drove in routine traffic. They developed abnormal heart rhythms and other signs of severe stress. Certain people—the "hot" reactors—respond to even ordinary annoyances in ways that bring on or worsen a wide variety of physical conditions. For instance, people living near airports visit their doctors more frequently, have many more physical complaints, and take more medications than do people living in quiet areas. In other words, stress itself isn't really dangerous; rather, how *you react* to stress may determine your emotional and physical well-being. Doctors now know that many physical problems—including hypertension, indigestion, headaches, asthma, colitis, peptic ulcers, and, according to many research scientists, even cancer—are stress-related. Foremost among stress-related conditions, however, is heart disease, which can be deadly.

5
The Deadly Triple Play

Analysis of stress responses has revealed three emotional traps that often cause prolonged and potentially deadly responses: the Sisyphus syndrome, emotional entrapment, and type A behavior. If you begin to recognize yourself in the descriptions of these traps, don't be overly alarmed. To some extent, these emotional land mines are part of nearly everyone's life; on some people, however, they have an especially powerful influence. Also, a "pure" picture of these types or situations is rare. Usually some characteristics overlap.

The Sisyphus Syndrome

The Sisyphus syndrome describes a combination of personality traits that can be lethal. Dr. Stuart Wolf and his colleagues coined this term, derived from the legendary king of Corinth who was condemned to Hades and given the endless task of rolling a huge stone up a mountain. Each time Sisyphus would reach the top, the stone would roll back down the mountain, and his labors would begin anew.

People with lots of Sisyphus traits joylessly and ceaselessly strive for difficult or unattainable goals, in both their work and their personal lives. Usually they have grown up in families where work was deemed all-important—the primary virtue and obligation. Often from a family with stern parents, people with Sisyphus traits learned the economic "facts of life" early, began work as youngsters, frequently have multiple jobs, and generally don't know how to enjoy the fruits of their labors. True workaholics, they define their entire lives by the work they do.

Dealing with people who rate high in Sisyphus traits is rarely pleasant—often bull-headed, they never take shortcuts and never "finesse" any project, no matter how big or small. They rarely delegate tasks, even when they aren't completely qualified to do something. No matter what, a Sisyphus will inflexibly and doggedly struggle with a project. This determination leads to a certain kind of underproductivity: A true Sisyphus can labor furiously at a project and yet not get the job done in a timely and efficient way. People with Sisyphus traits will labor even harder, their stress loads will mount, and they become victims of their own inflexibility.

A Sisyphus rarely recognizes personal limitations. The willingness to expend endless hours and maximum effort may gain this person a very demanding job and thus a reward for workaholic ways. Unfortunately, the catch is that the job often requires more education or experience than the Sisyphus really has, resulting in an unproductive struggle with a situation that is beyond his or her abilities. Unable to delegate authority or obtain help, the Sisyphus struggles harder, increasing the stress load even more.

People with Sisyphus traits have trouble enjoying themselves away from work, since their entire self-images depend on their work roles. They don't enjoy vacations because they only feel alive at work. But they don't truly enjoy work either, because their jobs lead to endless cycles of unproductive striving, frustration, discontent, and resentment.

People often think of the perfectionist hard-working Sisyphus type as a man who works endless hours at the office. But there are Sisyphus women too. The Sisyphus "superwoman" may be a homemaker; hers must be the cleanest and best-kept house; her meals must be the most varied, every dish made from scratch. Her kids must be the best dressed and the best behaved, and they must bring home the best grades. Today, with more women than ever before combining homemaking, working, and child care, women are exhibiting increased levels of Sisyphus traits. Such women may work the equivalent of two, three, or more jobs (wife, mother, homemaker, and career) and yet manage to accomplish none of them satisfactorily.

The Sisyphus man or woman rolls emotional boulders uphill endlessly. This mindset activates a prolonged fight-or-flight response throughout the body, which can have dire long-range consequences for the heart.

Al Tyrell had been employed by a printing company for many years. He worked on a press for long hours, earning a fine income. However, he might as well have been living in poverty: he and his wife never ate out, saw a movie only once or twice a year (at his wife's insistence), and had few friends and a meager social life. They led a constricted, one-dimensional life. For Al, life was all work.

Al grew up in New Jersey. He had his first job at age 8, working in an uncle's diner. By age 14, he was working twenty hours a week, in addition to attending school. As soon as he could, Al quit school and got a job. By age 20 he was married, and he and his wife had two children in two years. With bulldog tenacity, Al worked overtime, scrimping and saving for his children's future.

Over the years, Al became a skilled press operator, although he was such a perfectionist that he often needed extra time to get the job done. But he was a hard worker who gladly put in overtime (even on weekends), much to his wife's annoyance.

Even after his children graduated from college, Al worked as hard as ever. Spending less time than ever with family or friends, he was a confirmed workaholic even though he no longer had to scrimp for an undefined future. Work was simply his way of life.

Al's troubles began one year before we saw him as a patient, when he became line supervisor of the printing section. Now he was in charge of 32 people operating eight machines. Al's perfectionism got him into trouble. Overly involved in every detail of the presses—including machines that were more sophisticated than the one he had once operated—he got into deep water. Production demands increased, and Al couldn't find the time to master the technical details of the newer presses.

His relationships with his operators (all former coworkers) began deteriorating. They began voicing resentment at his need to check everything. Al's obstinacy meant that his operators had to work overtime to keep up with production schedules. Although overtime pay was good, the operators had no wish to work fifty or more hours each week.

One day Al, arguing heatedly with an operator about the best way to "run the next job through," felt a gripping pain in the middle of his chest. Clutching his chest, Al knew something was terribly wrong. He was rushed to the hospital and soon found himself in the coronary care unit with a heart attack.

Some weeks later, Al was back home, knowing that at age 48 he'd almost died of a heart attack. Something in his life would have to change if he wished to go on living.

The Sisyphus syndrome is more common than you may think. Most of us have some Sisyphus traits, and they can help make us successful. However, people whose entire makeup is dominated by Sisyphus traits are prone to developing heart disease. The following diagram demonstrates how this may happen:

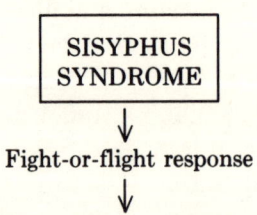

SISYPHUS SYNDROME
↓
Fight-or-flight response
↓
Increased nervous system response; outpouring of adrenaline; increased heart rate, increased blood pressure, increased serum lipids and cholesterol, increased platelet clumping and a tendency for blood to clot; coronary artery spasm
↓
Coronary artery narrowing with or without symptoms
↓
HEART ATTACK

The following questionnaire will pinpoint your Sisyphus traits. Be as honest with yourself as possible. If you have a genuine doubt about how to score a particular question, check the higher category.

	Often	Sometimes	Rarely
	(2 pts.)	(1 pt.)	(0 pts.)
1. Once I begin a book, I read it cover to cover, whether or not I like it.	____	____	____
2. By the second day of a vacation, I find myself thinking about returning to work.	____	____	____
3. I stick to my schedule for doing chores, no matter what.	____	____	____
4. I find myself involved in more projects than I can handle.	____	____	____
5. I find that the only one I can trust to do a job well is myself.	____	____	____
6. My day never seems to have enough hours.	____	____	____
7. I think about the next day's work in the middle of the night.	____	____	____
8. Approaching the end of one project, I immediately launch into the next one.	____	____	____
9. Although I work furiously, I'm not always sure at what I'm aiming.	____	____	____

	Often	Sometimes	Rarely
	(2 pts.)	(1 pt.)	(0 pts.)
10. I find praise from others difficult to accept.	___	___	___
11. I feel most fulfilled while I'm working.	___	___	___
12. I consider many of my colleagues lazy or unmotivated.	___	___	___
13. I get restless when I have a lot of free time.	___	___	___
14. When I reach a goal I had set for myself, I don't seem to be as satisfied as I thought I would be.	___	___	___
Add the scores for your total points	_____

How You Score

0-6 points: You have nothing to worry about. You rank low on Sisyphus traits. There are, however, other emotional land mines in life. Keep reading.

7-15 points: You rank moderately for Sisyphus traits. If you are on the lower range of the scale (closer to 7 points) you are controlling these traits; as you approach 15, you approach becoming a Sisyphus, and you may be prone to cardiovascular disease. Keep reading.

16-28 points: You are a true Sisyphus. You have many traits that can spell trouble for you and your heart. Keep reading. You need to know if you are bothered by other emotional life traps and, if so, to learn how to deal with them.

Emotional Entrapment

H. D. Thoreau once said: "The mass of men lead lives of quiet desperation." In a similar vein, emotional entrapment is the second great stumbling block of many people's lives, involving a frustrating and demoralizing situation or relationship from which there is no easy or acceptable way out. Such a situation can produce stress on a daily basis and eat away at your heart. Emotional entrapment that is easily recognizable (such as a bad marriage) is called *obvious entrapment*, and it can be a major source of ongoing stress and frustration.

Emotional entrapment can occur in less obvious ways, both at work and in one's personal life—a series of distressing little encounters in life, petty, nagging annoyances that lead to chronic resentment and stress. We call this *invisible entrapment*, a term borrowed from doctors Robert Eliot and Alan Forker, who coined it in an article in the *Journal of the American Medical Association*. Typically, victims feel obligated out of duty, guilt, or fear of offending to remain in situations they truly hate but cannot escape. An example would be someone's always feeling obligated to say "yes," even though he feels like saying "No!" This everyday entrapment can have many sources.

Although we often consider unfulfilled men such as Peter Fitzpatrick the primary victims of emotional entrapment, many working women are victims too. This life trap is thought to account in part for the increasing numbers of younger people (men *and* women) who now have symptoms of coronary artery disease. Statistics obtained during a ten-year study of the residents of Framingham, Massachusetts, show that certain women—secretaries, clerks, bookkeepers, and salespeople—had a 12 percent rate of heart disease, compared to an average of 7.8 percent among women in general. Women clerical workers who were married and also had children suffered an astounding 21.3 percent rate!

Follow-up questions with these women showed that many considered themselves victims of emotional entrapment, both obvious and invisible. They thought that their husbands and children made enormous emotional demands on them and that they were locked into frustrating no-win situations. They also described their bosses as unsupportive.

At the center of emotional entrapment is the feeling that you have lost the crucial element of control, either at work or in other situations. You can't win and you can't get out of the situation. Such a setting can become a potent emotional liability, leading to frustration, feelings of demoralization, and, in turn, a prolonged priming of the fight-or-flight response and a host of physical disturbances throughout the body.

Although heart disease may be the long-range consequence of emotional entrapment, you can learn to pinpoint and minimize both obvious and invisible entrapment in your life.

The following diagram illustrates how emotional entrapment can be a lethal bind:

EMOTIONAL ENTRAPMENT

Feelings of being trapped in a no-win situation or relationship
↓
Fight-or-flight response
↓
Increased nervous system response; outpouring of adrenaline; increased heart rate; increased blood pressure, increased serum lipids and cholesterol, increased platelet clumping, and a tendency for blood to clot; coronary artery spasm
↓
Coronary artery narrowing, with or without symptoms
↓
HEART ATTACK

Use the following questionnaire to determine the level of emotional entrapment in your personal and work life. As with the questionnaire about Sisyphus traits, if you are unsure how to answer an item, score it in the higher category.

	Often	Sometimes	Rarely
	(2 pts.)	(1 pt.)	(0 pts.)
1. I feel that I have very few choices in my life.	_____	_____	_____
2. I have trouble saying no to people.	_____	_____	_____
3. I find myself in social situations I'd rather not be in.	_____	_____	_____

	Often	Sometimes	Rarely
	(2 pts.)	(1 pt.)	(0 pts.)
4. I dread Mondays when I have to go back to work.	____	____	____
5. I wish I could explode, but the consequences would be too great.	____	____	____
6. I find myself thinking that I should have chosen a different career.	____	____	____
7. I wish I could begin all over again.	____	____	____
8. I feel that my job is frustrating and unrewarding.	____	____	____
9. I feel that I'm just pleasing other people, not myself.	____	____	____
10. When a salesperson pressures me, the persuasion is so hard to resist that I buy the item.	____	____	____
11. I find myself wishing I could tell someone off.	____	____	____
12. I find myself hoping that my children don't follow in my footsteps.	____	____	____
Add the scores for your total points		_____	

How You Score

0-6: You rate low on emotional entrapment. You have many options in your life and are not locked into a frustrating and unfulfilled bind.

7-12: You rate in the middle ground for emotional entrapment. In certain areas of your life you feel trapped. As you approach a score of 12, your entrapment level increases.

13+: You rate very high for emotional entrapment. The chances are that you are frustrated in both social and work areas of your life. You may be trapped in a setting that leaves you feeling hopeless—possibly producing serious consequences for your heart.

We are all victims of emotional entrapment to some extent. The extent to which you are trapped in no-win settings determines how much this bind can damage your well-being and your heart.

Type A Behavior

The term *type A behavior* is used to describe certain behavior patterns which make up our third emotional pitfall. The term was formulated and popularized by Doctors Meyer Friedman and Ray H. Rosenman, who published findings in 1959 that men with certain behavior patterns seemed to have two to three times the risk of heart attack as did those who were calmer, type B men.

A coronary-prone type A person aggressively strives to accomplish as much as possible in the least amount of time, regardless of any obstacle in his path. This impatience is called *time urgency* and is coupled with intense *competitiveness* and *free-floating hostility*.

Type A behavior is not simply these people's reactions to stress; rather, it is behavior they exhibit in both pleasant and unpleasant circumstances. The type A person experiences nearly every situation as though it were a challenge. Driving a car in traffic or trying to relax on a beach, a type A individual must push impatiently ahead, cannot relax, and must always "win."

If you're a type A person, you constantly strive to move forward. You always feel pressured. You are hasty, restless, tense, and competitive in almost any setting, work or pleasure. You tend to drive, work, eat, walk, talk, and do most things faster than other people; this time urgency is part of your very being. You become angry if someone keeps you waiting, or if the driver in front of you goes too slow. Your life is a nonstop carousel of competition, hostility, and haste. Friedman and Rosenman aptly labeled this behavior "hurry sickness."

Here is a roster of type A characteristics. Check those that apply to you. Again, if in doubt about a characteristic, check it.

- I have trouble sitting and doing nothing.
- I interrupt others when they talk. I hurry their speech by shaking my head or by saying, "Uh huh" as they talk.
- I rarely listen when someone talks; instead, I'm thinking about what I'll say next.
- I get very annoyed when I'm kept waiting.
- I eat quickly and leave the table right away.
- I often drum or tap my fingers.
- I always play to win, even in a game with kids.
- I'm frequently told by others to slow down and take it easy.
- I do most things with great intensity, as though life or death depended on it.
- I tend to curse often, even in ordinary conversation.
- I respond to a verbal challenge with hostility.
- I often feel angry for no particular reason.
- I can't let a comment pass—I need to respond to any form of hostility.
- I often try to do two or more things at once.

As you can see, a sense of time urgency, competitiveness, and free-floating hostility are at the core of type A behavior. If you checked off six or more of these behavior patterns, you have a great deal of type A behavior. You are especially prone to feeling angry, frustrated, and thwarted (leading to more anger); these feelings activate the fight-or-flight response throughout your body.

A word of caution is appropriate here. This roster involves a large and complicated group of behaviors. Almost anyone will have some of these characteristics; the key is whether *many* of them are *frequently* part of your behavior. No individual shows pure type A behavior; rather, most people are a mixture of type A and the less aggressive, calmer type B. To what extent you fall into either type is a matter of degree and of one pattern dominating the other.

Type A behavior has been touted by some people as being *the* source of stress-induced damage to the heart. In our view, type A behavior, though significant, is only part of the problem. Not all people with type A behavior develop heart disease, and many people who do not demonstrate this behavior *do* develop cardiovascular disease. In fact, many victims of emotional entrapment demonstrate behavior *opposite* to type A. They "grin and bear it," bottling up a smoldering, low-level anger that never really emerges into aggressive, or even assertive, behavior.

Here is how type A behavior can damage your heart:

```
        ┌──────────┐
        │  TYPE A  │
        │ BEHAVIOR │
        └──────────┘
   Rushing, hostility, frustration
                ↓
       Fight-or-flight response
                ↓
Prolonged physiologic cardiovascular changes wear away at your heart
                ↓
Coronary artery narrowing, with or without symptoms
                ↓
            HEART ATTACK
```

No one really knows why certain people develop type A behavior patterns. Dr. Friedman speculates that type A behavior may spring from a lack of unqualified love from parents during childhood—love was given only when the child was "good." In other words, love came to be viewed by the child as a reward. Remember, type A is not a so-called personality type, and it is not a psychiatric diagnosis; it is rather a group of coronary-prone behaviors that can lead to heart disease.

The Three Behaviors Combined

The Sisyphus syndrome, emotional entrapment, and type A behavior all describe unhealthy styles of thinking, feeling, and reacting to life stresses. They are a triple threat for heart disease. They often exist separately in different people. Even more deadly, they can occur in any one person in combination, with one or another predominating. When they are combined, the vicious cycle that results can be cumulative, doing even more damage to the heart. Here is how it works:

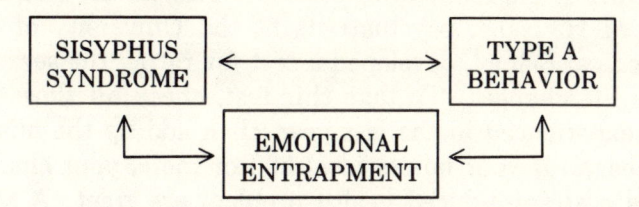

```
┌─────────────┐            ┌─────────────┐
│  SISYPHUS   │◄──────────►│   TYPE A    │
│  SYNDROME   │            │  BEHAVIOR   │
└─────────────┘            └─────────────┘
   ▲     └──►┌─────────────┐◄──┘    ▲
   └─────────│  EMOTIONAL  │────────┘
             │ ENTRAPMENT  │
             └─────────────┘
```

In a study of patients who demonstrated many Sisyphus traits combined with type A behavior, doctors were actually able to predict who eventually would have a heart attack! Imagine how much greater your risk of heart disease is if you rate high in type A behavior and Sisyphus traits *and* you are in a state of emotional entrapment.

Awareness of these emotional land mines has practical importance. If you recognize them as components of your own emotional landscape, you can change or modify them.

Major Life Changes

Awareness of these emotional variables is clearly important. Recognition of the importance of life changes and major stresses is also crucial. Most physicians believe that stress and your reaction to it play a central role in many illnesses, especially heart disease. A heart attack or the onset of coronary artery disease symptoms often follows a year of too many stressful events.

> Harry Fullman and his wife separated after thirty-five years of marriage. Harry had retired six months earlier, and the couple had moved to Florida. Harry's retirement and the increased time he spent with his wife strained an already-troubled marriage. The couple argued very frequently. Although they always had disagreements, Harry never thought them so serious that his wife would move out.
>
> Soon after his wife left, Harry began having chest pains. He visited his physician, who referred him to a cardiologist. After coronary angiography, the cardiologist recommended that

Harry undergo coronary bypass surgery. The combination of retirement and separation had proved too much for Harry. His heart paid the price.

To predict stress-related illnesses, Dr. Thomas H. Holmes and Dr. Richard H. Rahe, psychiatrists at the University of Washington Medical School, developed a test for rating the seriousness of various life changes. To take this test, check off those events you have experienced in the last year, then add up the numerical values of each. If your points total 300 or more, your chances of developing a stress-induced health problem are great. A score of 150 or more suggests that you should seriously consider how to reduce the stresses in your life. In a real sense, this test* is for everyone, whether a heart patient or not.

Event during the Past Year	*Score*
Death of spouse	100
Divorce	73
Marital separation	65
Jailing or institutionalization	63
Death of a close family member	63
Major injury or illness	53
Marriage	50
Fired from job	47
Marital reconciliation	45
Retirement	45
Major change in health or behavior of family member	44
Pregnancy	40
Sexual difficulties	39
Gaining a new family member	39
Major business change (merger, bankruptcy)	39
Major change in financial status	38
Death of a close friend	37
Changing to a different line of work	36
Major change in frequency of arguments with spouse	35
Mortgage or loan for major purchase	31
Foreclosure	30
Major work change	29

*The Social Readjustment Rating Scale; Journal of Psychosomatic Research; 2;213 (1967)

Event during the Past Year	Score
Departure of child from home	29
Trouble with in-laws	29
Outstanding personal achievement	28
Spouse starting or stopping job	26
Start or end of school	26
Major change in living conditions	25
Change in personal habits	24
Trouble with boss	23
Major change in working hours or conditions	20
Change in residence	20
New school	20
Major change in recreation	19
Major change in church activities	19
Major change in social activities	18
Mortgage or loan for lesser purchase	17
Major change in sleeping habits	16
Major change in number of family get-togethers	15
Major change in eating habits	15
Vacation	13
Christmas	12
Minor legal violations (traffic tickets, etc.)	11
Total	_____

Clearly, some events are major life crises. Others, such as changing to a different line of work or changing one's residence, are important life changes that do not have a crisis element. Still others are the stuff of everyday life—vacation, the Christmas holiday, getting a traffic ticket.

Let's look at Harry Fullman's score and see how he does on this stress test.

Event	Score
Harry and his wife separated.	65
Harry had just retired.	45
Harry's financial status changed.	38
The frequency of Harry's arguments with his wife changed.	35
The Fullmans moved to Florida.	20
Total	203

Harry Fullman's score is well above 150, but less than the 300 score that may be an indicator of a forthcoming illness. We don't know if Harry obtained a mortgage for his new home in Florida (another 31 points); we don't know if a close friend died (another 37 points) or if Harry's church and social activities changed (37 more points). It's a good bet that these last two changes did occur, since Harry and his wife moved a thousand miles away from their former home. Most likely, the closer we look at Harry's life setting, the closer he'll get to the 300 mark.

Thus, in addition to everyday stresses, you must cope with major life events that require additional adaptation. These stresses can feed into an already overloaded system and help bring on heart disease or other illnesses.

6
Heart Attack: The Ultimate Challenge

Charles Russo was trudging through the snowy streets of Stamford, Connecticut, when he suddenly felt a gripping pain in his chest. "It felt like someone was sitting on the middle of my chest," he said later. "The pain was crushing. It even went down to my elbows."

Charles felt faint and within moments began sweating profusely, even though the temperature had dipped to 20 degrees. Realizing that something was dreadfully wrong, he stumbled up the stairs of his house and rang the bell. Within 15 minutes he was in a hospital coronary care unit (CCU).

Charles Russo was lucky. He realized that he was having a heart attack or at least that something was seriously wrong. Above all, he didn't delay. One important reason that people die of heart attacks is that they delay getting to a hospital. Many people have trouble admitting to themselves that something serious is actually happening to them. Some cannot believe that their hearts are involved; others attribute their discomfort to gas or an intestinal upset. Even people who *know* that they have heart disease tend to delay, perhaps thinking that their attacks are just another episode of angina that will soon pass. Oddly, a recent visit to a physician often makes people delay, probably because a stamp of good health from the doctor gave them a false sense of security.

Procrastination in the face of cardiac symptoms can be fatal. As a matter of fact, the majority of deaths from coronary heart disease occur *before* patients get to a hospital. You must know the cardinal warning signals of a heart attack:

- The first warning is an uncomfortable sense of pressure, fullness, squeezing, or pain in the center of your chest (usually beneath the breastbone) that lasts more than a few minutes.
- The pain may spread to (or be experienced only in) the shoulders, arms, elbows, or jaw. The pain may seem to be nothing more than an upset stomach. Figure 4 illustrates typical pain intensity and location.
- The pain may grow more severe and may be coupled with dizziness, fainting, sweating, or shortness of breath. All or some of these signals may occur, and they may be accom-

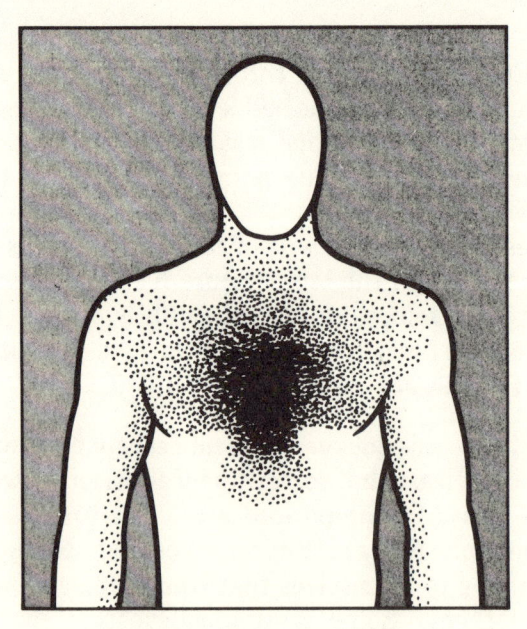

Intensity and Location of Pain

Figure 4.

panied by severe anxiety or a sense of dread and impending doom.

Many people have full-blown heart attacks with minimal symptoms (the so-called silent heart attack) and never know they went through it. The danger in such a situation is that they may suffer a second—possibly fatal—heart attack.

Why a Heart Attack May be Fatal

A heart attack, or myocardial infarction, is the death of heart muscle that occurs when a coronary artery is completely blocked. Although part of the heart muscle is destroyed, usually plenty of healthy muscle remains to continue to pump blood to support life.

On very rare occasions, a heart attack may be so massive—destroying a very large portion of heart tissue—that the heart can no longer pump effectively, causing shock or heart failure. This is usually fatal.

More often, the cause of death in a fatal heart attack is a disturbance in the heart's electrical activity. The heart has a built-in electrical network that keeps it contracting in a regular and rhythmic way. If this network is damaged, the heart's rhythmic pumping may be interrupted or become erratic. The heart may stop beating (cardiac arrest), or it may fibrillate (an irregular twitching motion). In either situation, the heart cannot pump effectively, and the body is deprived of oxygen and vital nutrients.

An attack is fatal if the heart's inability to pump effectively goes on for more than a few minutes. The brain (along with the rest of the body) is deprived of oxygen when the heart has shut down, and the brain is extremely sensitive to such deprivation.

Sudden Cardiac Death

Some people die suddenly when their hearts' electrical systems malfunction. The heart begins to quiver uselessly (fibrillation), and death occurs quickly. Sudden cardiac death may be the very first manifestation of heart disease for some unfortunate people—many do not actually have heart attacks. What happened? In many cases, stress is probably the cause.

At times of intense emotional stress, coronary artery spasm may occur. Chest pains caused by this spasm can be so frightening that the person may then have a full-blown panic attack. Some people may have lethal panic attacks without either chest pain or coronary artery spasm.

Excessive stimulation of the body by the supercharged, panic-struck mind can trigger fatal abnormal heart rhythms. An enormous outpouring of adrenaline into the bloodstream overstimulates the heart, as happened to the man who learned that his wife had died. This was lethal emotional stress.

Several possible causes of erratic heart rhythms can lead to sudden cardiac death:

- Coronary artery spasms can lead to panic, then to fibrillation.
- Coronary artery spasms can cause an inadequate blood supply to the heart's electrical system.
- A heart attack may damage tissue that contains the heart's electrical network, leading to fibrillation.
- Severe panic alone can trigger fibrillation and lead to death. (Some physicians think that people who suddenly die of emotional flooding may have built-in heart abnormalities.)

Panic can be a deadly enemy. It can occur at any time, but it often strikes heart attack victims when they are most vulnerable, before they get to a hospital. A heart attack can be a terrifying experience, causing panic and then cardiac arrhythmia. Even if no heart irregularity develops, panic prevents people from thinking and acting properly; it can lead to a delay in getting help, which can be lethal. To avoid the possibility of sudden cardiac death, know the body's warning signals and know what to do if you think you are having a heart attack.

What to Do If You Think You Are Having a Heart Attack

Heart attacks may begin during strenuous exertion, but most do not. There is no general rule about where or when symptoms begin. If you experience any of the symptoms we have described, *get to a hospital without delay.*

Don't worry about a false alarm. It's better to be a little embarrassed than to delay and risk deadly consequences. You will be happy to be told at the hospital that you are not having a heart attack.

The time between the onset of symptoms and the arrival at a hospital can be terrifying. Making the trip with a family member or friend (you should not be driving) will help. If you go in an ambulance, take a family member along with you. Having someone familiar with you will reduce the sense of strangeness and isolation that an ambulance with its screaming siren, a crowded emergency room, or a cardiac care unit may evoke. At such a time, having someone close can be a very powerful antidote to panic! You must do everything you can to counteract feelings of helplessness, anxiety, or panic.

At an emergency room you will be examined, you will have an electrocardiogram taken, and certain blood tests will be done. If the data indicate you may be having a heart attack, you will be admitted to the CCU. A definite diagnosis is often difficult to make in the first few hours.

About the CCU

The CCU is a section of the hospital used for treating patients who may be having a heart attack. CCUs are staffed by specially trained nurses and afford the utmost in protection against the possible complications of a heart attack (heart failure, cardiac arrest, or an irregular heart rhythm). A CCU can be a strange and frightening place to someone unfamiliar with its purpose and equipment. However, for some patients, the CCU is a comfortable and safe place, because they know they are being watched carefully.

When taken to a CCU, you will rest in bed, most likely in a private room. An intravenous infusion (IV) will be inserted into a vein of your arm, ensuring instant access to your bloodstream should emergency medication be needed. Small electrodes will be attached to your chest; they lead to a heart monitor (which looks like a small television) at your bedside. The image on the bedside monitor also appears on a screen at the central nursing station.

This sophisticated technology monitors your heart to see how it works. In many CCUs the information obtained is analyzed by a computer. Any change or abnormality that registers on the monitor triggers an alarm, and the staff is instantly alerted.

Most patients are aware that they are in the CCU because of the possibility of sudden death from a fatal arrhythmia. The actual risk is relatively low. A patient who makes it to the hospital has an excellent chance of recovering and returning to a normal life. Most serious problems occur within the first 24 hours and can be treated with medication or electrical stimulation of the heart.

A dangerous enemy during this crucial first day after a heart attack is anxiety, which can lead to panic and its effects on the heart. The heart-mind connection is vitally important here; your treatment must be directed toward your mind as well as your heart. This means keeping anxiety to a minimum. Tranquilizers are standard therapy.

Reducing Anxiety

Keep in mind that the CCU's primary purpose is to protect you. Sick people frequently feel that their lives have suddenly spun out of control and that they no longer have a say in what happens to them; doctors, nurses, even fate, seem to have assumed control over their lives. Feeling this way can lead some patients to think that stoic silence is the only way to handle illness, even when they are terrified.

Nothing could be farther from the truth! If you begin feeling upset or anxious, inform the CCU staff. *You* are the first line of defense against anxiety and its possible effects. Talking with the staff about anxiety helps, and you will be given medication (a tranquilizer) if necessary. This will help you feel calm and more in control. A sense that you have some control over events frequently will help to minimize your anxiety. Asking for and receiving a little reassurance at a bad moment can work wonders.

Visits from close family members while you are in the CCU are vital. These visits help to cut down on feelings of strangeness and isolation. Seeing a familiar face can be very important.

Today, hospitals recognize that the CCU environment should be pleasant and reassuring. Most are brightly colored places where each patient has a view from a window and there is sufficient sensory stimulation to avoid feelings of isolation and helplessness. Visiting is encouraged, and supportive contact with nurses and doctors is usually the rule.

Every patient will have an individual reaction to having a heart attack and being in a CCU. Usually, preexisting personality tendencies determine this. Despite differences among people, certain themes emerge with many patients.

After the first few days (when there is the greatest potential for anxiety) most patients realize that they are going to survive. This realization of course brings a feeling of relief, but along with the good feelings may come worry about the extent of cardiac damage and how it will affect their lives. At this time, some patients will feel depressed and will worry about the future. A physician's reassurance is crucial. Most patients feel genuinely reassured when their doctors tell them—truthfully—that they will be able to return to work, exercise, sex, and a full life after they leave the hospital.

It is also helpful to know that you have much more control over anxiety than you may think. By talking with the CCU staff about *any* uncomfortable feelings (emotional or physical), you enhance the probability of a speedy and uneventful recovery.

7

Beyond the CCU: Adjusting to New (and Not-So-Bad) Realities

Learning that you have any form of heart disease will certainly produce an emotional reaction. Naturally, if you have had a heart attack and have been in a CCU, your concerns will be more urgent than if you recently developed mild angina. If you've been diagnosed as having angina pectoris, you may worry that you will soon have a heart attack.

A diagnosis of heart disease must be taken seriously, but you have not been handed a death sentence. Nor have you been assigned a life of diminishing returns. You have had a brush with your own mortality, which is sobering, but you must now face a real challenge. That challenge is to live your life to the fullest while making certain important changes in the way you live.

The one supremely grave danger in dealing with heart disease is *fear*—fear of worsening your illness, fear of the future, fear of living your life. Fear is the stuff of invalidism.

Nearly every patient who develops heart disease has a variety of anxious concerns. These worries often take the form of questions; sometimes they are asked openly, sometimes less directly. Wondering how heart disease will change your life is normal.

Common Concerns

You may be worried about dying: How long will I live? Can I make long-range plans? Will I have another heart attack? If so, will it be fatal? What will become of my wife? My husband? My family? Your spouse may worry about the possibility of your dying. These are only some of the questions about death and dying that our patients ask.

Let's face it. Any illness can cause anxiety because of the real or threatened damage it may do to the body. This anxiety is realistic, but it must be kept in perspective. Actually, the risk of dying is small for most patients. Heart disease does carry the threat of bodily damage or death, but patients' fears often outweigh the realistic dangers. As we discussed in Chapter 1, people often consider the heart the very center of a person, the one indispensable part, the soul and very essence of a person. Most people regard the heart with an awestruck reverence reinforced by our daily expressions and folklore. The idea of the heart is imbued with so many meanings that, for many people, any heart problem becomes a highly charged issue that brings inordinate fear. In fact, once a patient recovers from a heart attack, the prognosis for a fulfilling and active life is excellent.

Insecurity about work is common. Will I be able to earn a living? Am I getting too old? If I get back to work will I be able to handle the job? Will I be an invalid? What about my future?

Other concerns involve the general quality of life. Will I have to give up delicious food? Am I falling apart? How will my family and friends relate to me? Can I drive a car? Can I drink a beer? Have a glass of wine? What about my sex life? Will I ever feel I'm normal? Will I have to forfeit all of life's pleasures?

We regularly see patients with all these concerns. Of course, different people deal with these worries in vastly different ways. Some respond to the life challenge quite well; others do not. Some patients who develop heart disease simply quit living.

> Daniel Weston, a 47-year-old school teacher, developed severe angina. After coronary angiography, he was advised to have coronary bypass surgery. The operation was done in short order. From that point on, Daniel's life changed completely.

Previously an energetic man, he was suddenly afraid to engage in any activities. Although he now had no symptoms of angina, Daniel feared that the least stress or activity would precipitate a fatal heart attack. He began insulating himself from everything.

We saw Daniel Weston in consultation when he applied for SSI (supplemental security income) because he felt he was disabled and could no longer work. Daniel's functional cardiac capacity, assessed by treadmill exercise testing, was normal; nevertheless he was totally disabled because he *believed* that he was! He didn't even have symptoms! Among other things, Daniel said:

I don't think you understand my fear. I'm afraid to get up out of a chair and walk across the room. I can imagine the pain starting up again, and then I can almost *feel* a crushing sensation in my chest ... and then the dizziness. I keep thinking that the slightest thing will cause a heart attack. That if I do anything, I'll end up in the hospital. And even if I don't die, I'll be a cripple.

Unfortunately, Daniel Weston was already a cripple. He had retreated from life. His invalidism was emotional.

John Mason, a physician, had a similar reaction. He suffered a heart attack; some months later, he was doing well. One year later, he developed angina and then underwent a bypass operation. He went back to work, but soon felt unable to continue with his practice. Each time he examined a patient, he was reminded of his own disease, and soon he could no longer tolerate treating patients with heart problems—it hit too close to home.

Curtailing his practice, he spent a great deal of time thinking about his own case, imagining pains in his chest. He became so obsessed with his "illness" that he could think of little else. His wife told us that he would sit for hours taking his blood pressure and checking his pulse. Then, placing the stethoscope over his heart, he would listen "for something."

When we saw him in consultation, clearly he was morbidly hypochondriacal and was suffering from a deep depression.

These cases are examples of patients who did poorly after learning they had heart disease. Their problems, however, did not reflect physical causes. Again, with occasional exceptions, heart disease rarely results in true physical disability!

Years ago, the medical profession had little to offer anyone with heart disease besides a rocking chair and the advice to "take it easy." Much less was known about the causes and treatment of heart disease, and many thought that heart patients had to "preserve" their weakened and damaged hearts. This approach, although well-intentioned, often led patients and those around them to believe that they were total or partial invalids.

Unfortunately, this misguided notion has lingered in the popular mind and in some segments of the medical community. As a consultant for a state bureau of Disability Determinations, one of the authors regularly sees heart patients whose only true disability is emotional! The patient, family, and even the doctors believe that the patient is a cripple. They are right, but the disability is emotional. Tragically, an army exists of people whose lives orbit about the notion of being disabled, and they are no longer productive members of society. They collect disability checks from the government or insurance companies. No matter how we try to encourage these people to come "back to life," they continue to retreat from a full life and all its pleasures.

In his book, *The Healing Heart* (Norton, 1983), Norman Cousins describes having to virtually rebel against his well-intentioned physicians to begin a regimen of rehabilitation after his heart attack. Becoming a "heart patient" did not make Mr. Cousins view himself as disabled. Rather, he refused to be victimized by emotional incapacitation.

Cousins points out that the body has its own natural tendency toward healing, if the proper emotional and physical conditions prevail. We agree completely. Given sufficient time, the blood vessels supplying the heart, even though severely narrowed or blocked, form a rich network of auxiliary vessels over the heart, making the tissue less vulnerable to being choked off by inadequate blood supply. These newly formed vessels are *collaterals* and are a product of the body's own restorative and survival mechanisms.

Cousins details how blocking out negative emotional reactions—such as severe anxiety, depression, and panic—is essential for healing and restoration. He demonstrates how proper diet, exercise, and the fostering of healthy, optimistic, and positive feelings can be harnessed for healing. Following his massive heart attack, Norman Cousins reoriented certain stress-related aspects of his life so successfully that he virtually began a new career. Henry Kissinger and Alexander Haig are two more of the many people who have continued with highly successful careers despite coronary heart disease serious enough to require bypass surgery.

We will show you how to deal successfully with heart disease, no matter how compromised your coronary arteries may now be. Ultimately, your body and mind can work together for healing and restoration. You must allow these mechanisms to flourish so that you can adapt to the changes and challenges that heart disease invokes.

PART 2

Heartplan: A Step-by-Step Strategy for Physical and Emotional Well-Being

Introduction

Emotional factors, crucial in bringing on heart disease, are vital in any recovery program. They must be considered along with the physical aspects of your program for health and well-being. Heartplan is our comprehensive, step-by-step strategy for dealing with heart disease to benefit your heart and allow you a full and active life. With or without heart disease, it should be exciting to wake up each morning and begin a new day.

Heartplan is divided into steps; not every step applies to each reader. You may have had a heart attack, or you may have angina pectoris or hypertension. Your plan may be slightly different in these different instances. If you do not have heart disease and wish to avoid it completely, you can benefit enormously from what follows. Heartplan is organized so that readers can use the steps that apply to their individual situations.

Step 1: Setting New Priorities and Realistic Goals

A physician friend of ours (we'll call him Dr. Striver) was very well known in the profession and was considered tops in his specialty. Barely a day passed without his telephone ringing off the hook, and his consultation schedule was so busy that new patients had to wait six to eight weeks for an appointment.

Besides his consulting work, he was on staff at a major hospital and on the faculty of a prestigious medical school. His days began at 7:00 a.m. and usually ended near midnight. Office patients, hospital rounds, conferences, committee meetings, lectures, seminars, fund-raisers, medical society meetings, radio and television appearances, and magazine interviews were some of his commitments.

Then he became ill with pneumonia. It was a serious illness; his fever went up to 104 degrees, and for a while his life was in jeopardy. Fortunately, after a long period of therapy, he recovered completely. But he'd paid a price. Dr. Striver, a vigorous, robust, middle-aged man, had lost 35 pounds and was a withered version of his former self.

Recuperation was long and arduous but successful. Seven months after his illness, he was back at the office seeing one or two patients each day. He was not yet strong enough to return to his hospital and medical school obligations, but no one doubted that he would soon return to normal.

Months later, we were surprised to learn that he'd pared down his staff to one secretary and a nurse. Even though he had not yet returned to his other activities, we were still certain that he would soon come roaring through the medical center doors and the whirlwind would begin anew.

More than a year after his illness began, Dr. Striver had still not returned to his former activities. He had "faded away" from the medical scene, and everyone wondered why. True, he'd attended one session of grand rounds (a weekly hospital staff meeting at which a challenging case is presented), and he'd appeared healthy and attentive. He seemed contemplative as he listened to the case history unfold. Not his usual self, he hadn't shot from his seat with an instant diagnosis, nor had he peppered the presenting physicians with his usual array of challenging and provocative questions. We wondered what had happened.

Soon afterward, Dr. Striver telephoned us to refer a patient for evaluation. He said that this patient seemed to have emotional problems, even though his symptoms were chest pains. Would this patient be a good candidate for counseling? Involved in writing this book, we were "primed" for such a case.

After seeing the patient, we telephoned Dr. Striver to discuss the case. During our talk we mentioned how we missed the occasional hallway encounter with him at the medical center and made plans to meet for lunch the following week.

Our lunch meeting was profoundly revealing. Dr. Striver said that he'd curtailed his practice to a fraction of its former size. He was now seeing fewer patients and spending more time with each one, even asking about their emotional lives! He'd discovered a new interest in the psychological aspects of physical symptoms and was planning to attend a series of conferences dealing with this fascinating subject.

Dr. Striver had changed other things in his life as well. He and his wife attended the opera together, although for years his wife had gone with a friend because the doctor was too busy. They began going to movies, concerts, and restaurants, and were planning a trip to Mexico. In addition, they had rented a weekend cottage where the trout fishing was reputed to be excellent. He'd rekindled an old love for fishing, which he'd relinquished upon entering medical school.

Clearly, our friend was not the same person he'd been before his illness. Here was a man whose life had been a nonstop carousel of frantic medical activity; his workaholic ways had saturated his very being. In contrast, Dr. Striver was now more reflective and less intense. He enjoyed new delights, involving himself with films, theater, opera, and psychology, and was about to reactivate a boyhood pleasure. In all this, he seemed to feel a sense of adventure in rediscovering long-lost positive feelings in both himself and the world around him. Clearly he and his wife were redefining their lives together.

Amazed at this transition from a true Sisyphus syndrome type (with some type A behavior) to a reflective person who seemed to know what he wanted out of life, we asked how he'd accomplished this remarkable transformation.

"After I got out of the hospital, I asked myself what I *really* wanted from life," said Dr. Striver. "It seemed that I'd been working harder and harder for reasons that were totally beyond me, as though work had somehow become an end in itself."

He explained how he'd set about reordering his priorities and goals after his illness. He now possessed some inkling of the preciousness of life. He realized that he'd lost perspective on what place work should have in the fabric of his life. Work, he decided, should provide some pleasure by itself, but there's got to be more. Work should allow him to experience other meaningful pleasures. Reflecting about his life and goals, he realized that he'd been blindly pursuing an illusory vision of happiness, one that was little more than a vague and receding horizon he'd never seemed able to grasp.

After explaining how he decided that a total revamping of his life-style and priorities was in order, he sat back and gazed upward. "It's funny," he said bemusedly. "When I realized that my life was consumed by trivia, with worries about committee meetings or grand rounds, or some other nonsense, I realized that to determine quickly if something is really important to me, I need only ask myself one simple question. *Is this worth dying for?*"

Dr. Striver's case illustrates important points. Many people who have had a brush with death can put their lives into a more sensible perspective. A periodic review of your goals and priorities is probably helpful, no matter what your situation. It is essential when you have heart disease.

Unfortunately, many patients with coronary heart disease have an abundance of Sisyphus traits. Their workaholic ways have permeated their lives, robbing them of pleasure in most areas of life. As Dr. Striver said, it's as though work and its daily details have somehow become ends in themselves. For many, life becomes little more than an endless exercise in joyless striving and toil. Exactly what are these people chasing?

When we ask these patients what they really want in their lives, they cannot tell us. We hear a variety of abstract answers: success, happiness, fulfillment, security. And so it goes. Oddly, very few people answer Contentment.

We ask these patients, "What could you possibly acquire or accomplish that would make you happy? Secure? Fulfilled?

Successful? A befuddled look then comes over them. They stammer for a moment, pause, reflect, mumble something, and then seem lost in thought. Soon, they shake their heads and look exasperated. The truth is, when asked what they truly want, they don't know!

Many seek some poorly defined and abstract idea, a fantasy of what they think will make them happy. If they manage to obtain it (whatever it is), they then long for the next thing, which, of course, is beyond their grasp. Engaged in this quest for something they haven't really defined, they live a life of chronic discontent, which inevitably leads to disappointment and frustration.

Life, by its very nature, is filled with challenges. It is occasionally disappointing, often difficult to fathom, and never without problems. We don't always get exactly what we want. Only by coming to terms with these facts of life can we feel reasonably content. Rolling emotional boulders uphill in a joyless Sisyphus-like quest for unattainable or poorly defined goals will set into motion the dangerous physical reactions that can lead to and worsen heart disease. Clearly, also, the Sisyphus orientation guarantees feelings of disillusionment.

Resetting certain priorities and goals is vital, as Dr. Striver discovered. Don't abandon ambition or excitement; don't rationalize failure or content yourself with mediocrity. Resetting priorities simply means taking "time out for life" and reorienting yourself, defining and setting goals that are realistic and attainable.

Few people question their life priorities and goals. Naturally, it is better to think about these issues without having to deal with heart disease and its possible consequences.

The next few pages pose certain questions. Trying to answer them can increase your awareness of your goals and key you into changing any that may be unrealistic, poorly defined, or disproportionately meaningful in your life. Answer these questions as forthrightly as possible. Some may seem simple, but reflecting on them will help you look more deeply into yourself.

1. *Is this worth dying for?*

As Dr. Striver discovered, this question can quickly set a variety of burning issues into proper perspective. It requires that you consider what things are truly important to you. Ask yourself: Is this promotion, this single customer, this account, this project, this appointment, this sale, this report, this 7:00 a.m. flight, this membership in this country club so truly important? Is it worth losing sleep over? Am I willing to place stress and strain on my heart and risk the possible long-run consequences of coronary heart disease?

Remember, after overcoming his illness Dr. Striver had a healthy heart; he never even developed heart disease. For someone with heart disease, whether something is worth dying for becomes an even more meaningful measure, since undue stress itself aggravates, and even causes, coronary heart disease.

2. Am I striving for goals that are poorly defined and unrealistic?

This is a difficult question; to answer it you must take a long, hard look at your goals, opportunities, and limitations.

Ask: What are my goals for the day? For the week? For the next month? Six months? For the next year? Beyond? Can I put my goals—both work and personal—into words, or are they abstractions that have little true meaning? Beware of one-word goals such as *happiness* and *success*. Why do I wish to attain these goals? What will happen if I do not reach them? Another way to examine your personal and work goals is to ask yourself if anything in your life would truly change were you to win the state lottery?

To explore your opportunities, ask: Do I truly have opportunities in my work, or am I waging an uphill and inevitably losing battle? Can I create opportunities without feeding into my Sisyphus traits? What are my realistic chances for promotion? For getting the next big account? A salary increase? The next juicy assignment? Can I define my best qualities—both business and personal?

Assessing your limitations can include these questions: Am I as good as I think I am at what I do? Have I learned all I can about my work? Do others do what I do better? If so, what makes them better? Can I improve my own standing without getting caught up in a Sisyphus frenzy? Do I know my shortcomings, both business and personal?

3. Have I substituted material accomplishments (or their pursuit) for the more personal and human rewards in my life?

Answering this question involves a host of others: Has my work overshadowed my marriage? My relationships with my children? My friends? Do I ever take a truly nonbusiness vacation? Do I have moments of genuine satisfaction, especially when I'm away from work? Can I look forward to taking periodic miniretreats (such as three-day weekends) with someone I love? Is there anyone in my life to whom I can tell my deepest fears and confide my deepest wishes? Is sex with my partner rich, fun, and spontaneous?

4. *Have I sought out constant, ungratifying activity to avoid introspection? When I am introspective, is it painful?*

Introspection raises some of these issues: When was the last time I thought about loving and caring? Do I think about relationships and what they mean to me? Do I ever wonder if I can improve various nonwork parts of my life? Do I question myself?

5. *Will I allow my partner to help me reassess and rearrange my priorities?*

So you may see that a confirmed Sisyphus type can change his ways, let's look at the following case:

Frank Barker was a 51-year-old business executive when he had his heart attack. A true workaholic who rated very high in Sisyphus traits, he found himself reassessing his life's priorities during his recuperation. His brush with death was a sobering experience for Frank; once out of the CCU, he became painfully aware of how his business activities encroached into every area of his life. Still in the hospital, feeling alone and frightened, Frank realized how-one dimensional his life had become.

Frank's most troubling realization involved his relationship with his wife: The one leisure activity Frank and his wife shared was their membership in a tennis club. But when Frank examined his activities there, he could see that here too he was all work. The club was a hotbed of business activity; barely a weekend passed when Frank did not play doubles with an assortment of high-powered business cronies. Tennis was secondary. Business was discussed on the court, in the locker room, and at dinner. Frank's wife might as well have been absent. Frank realized that his wife had long ago become a silent and barely visible backdrop to his own extended business activities at the club. Frank was constantly wheeling and dealing. His days—even at the tennis club—were a frantic course of nonstop bargaining and deal making.

A few days after getting out of the CCU, Frank asked his wife if she was happy with their arrangement at the tennis club. She gently told him how alienated from him she felt not only at the club, but in their lives in general. For the first time in years, Frank and his wife talked about their marriage. They discussed their lives' directions, both as individuals and as a couple. After some very painful soul-searching, Frank decided that he had to rearrange certain priorities. And he would make these changes only after talking about them with his wife.

In what became a new "era" for the couple, the Barkers decided to spend more time genuinely together. They gave up their membership in the tennis club and joined another where Frank knew no one and had no business connections. Playing tennis together, the Barkers established a truly social basis for their weekends. Frank Barker and his wife began to reassess other priorities in their life together and continued to make important and positive changes.

Interestingly, Frank informed us that his business didn't suffer because he limited his work strictly to business hours—which he decreased.

If you rate high in Sisyphus traits, you must review your work habits and assess the results they yield. Frank Barker's experience is not unusual; cutting down on certain work activities did not diminish his business. If anything, he became more efficient. As Frank Barker did, you can learn to *work smarter, not harder*.

We have found that certain questions can help you assess the results you are now getting from your present work habits. These simple questions can help you focus on issues that you may normally take for granted:

1. Am I working as efficiently as I can?
2. If I work fewer hours, will my job, income, or status suffer?
3. If I work harder, will I get more? If so, more what? Money? Privilege? Prestige? Fame? Security?
4. If I do get more of whatever I want, what will I do with it?

5. If I could get *one* more thing out of work (money, increased status, seniority, benefits, vacation time, admiration of my colleagues, etc.) what would it be? If I work longer hours, including weekends, will I get this one additional thing?
6. Could I accomplish the same amount of work in less time, without rushing and without doing a patchwork job?

Frank Barker and Dr. Striver have something in common. In reevaluating their priorities, both men cut back on the incredible amount of time and energy they spent at work. Both expanded other important spheres of their lives—their relationships with their loved ones and their social lives. Both men realized that, busy as they'd been, their lives were truly constricted and one-dimensional before their illnesses. Each then went on to expand and enrich his life in various ways once this realization hit home.

Norman Cousins, in *The Healing Heart*, eloquently describes how he became more aware of life around him after his heart attack. He discovered that his senses were heightened: Fragrances seemed more aromatic; colors seemed brighter and deeper. The sights and sounds and feelings of life became more meaningful, precious, and beautiful. Many of our patients have described similar experiences. Once they take stock of themselves and their lives, many people can use the life crisis of heart disease as an opportunity to change, to grow, to heighten intimacy with their partners, and to find a deeper appreciation of the good things in thier lives.

Take time out for life. Harness the same mental energies that have contributed to your heart disease and redirect them toward new and healthier attitudes and ways of living.

Don't wait until you are in a CCU recovering from a heart attack to seriously reassess your life's goals and priorities. If you have developed angina pectoris or if you wish to avoid heart disease, the time to begin is now. The rest of your life awaits you!

Step 2: Decreasing Both Obvious and Invisible Emotional Entrapment

To some extent, we are all victims of life traps that cause us emotional and physical distress. Any society assigns its members certain roles and duties. No one is completely free of burdensome obligations, and everyone occasionally feels frustrated and trapped.

This step will help you determine if you have important emotional traps in your personal and work life. If you do, you can change these arrangements (or your view of them) so that you feel less mired in heart-damaging binds that can make you miserable and compromise your health.

Conquering Obvious Entrapment

Entrapment often takes an obvious form such as feeling suffocated in an unhappy marriage, relationship, or job. The entrapment is usually obvious to the sufferer (and to everyone else) and can bring on emotional pain and stress-induced illness. The following case is an example of obvious entrapment taken from our practices.

Richard Michaels was a 48-year-old administrator of a government agency. Over the years, he had been a real dynamo (Sisyphus traits mixed with type A behavior) and had transformed a sluggish, mediocre agency into a fast-paced, streamlined operation. But then things spun out of his control. Policy changes made by high government officials affected Richard's agency, and Richard was informed that his bureau would be slowly phased out. His seniority guaranteed him a fine salary until retirement, and there was no danger of his being unemployed; the danger for Richard was a different kind.

At 48, Richard realized that he presided over an almost-defunct agency. Things would eventually grind to a weary halt. Locked in and frustrated, Richard watched helplessly as his hard-won accomplishments began draining away. His staff was reduced by attrition (retirements and transfers), and Richard hated going to the office each morning. He felt useless and demoralized. No challenge was left at work, and Richard found it hard to feel good about anything, but Richard could not quit. To quit would mean looking for a job outside of government—at age 48, a difficult task. A transfer would lose him his seniority. With no control over his situation, Richard Michaels was a helpless victim of a major life entrapment.

Some months later, while shoveling snow in front of his house, Richard felt a dull pain in the center of his chest. It subsided when he rested. The pain returned several times over the next few days, and Richard finally visited his physician. The diagnosis was made—angina pectoris. Richard's angina was mild; it came on only when he exerted himself, and rest or a nitroglycerine tablet promptly relieved the pain. Angiography indicated that his coronary arteries were not dangerously narrowed, but he did have atherosclerosis.

Medical treatment helped, but Richard's angina pains soon took on a disturbingly clear pattern; they got worse each time he went to the office. Richard sought psychological counseling, not because of his chest pains, but because he'd become increasingly depressed over his work situation. The fact that he had a heart condition further demoralized him.

In a couple of sessions, the source of Richard's problems became obvious. We discussed his job, asking him to enumerate the various aspects of his work that he used to enjoy and find rewarding. Wistfully Richard described what he'd liked at work: managing people, requesting financial appropriations, and solving organizational snags.

Once Richard had accurately named these enjoyable work activities, a very simple practical question arose. How might he find a situation where he could apply these skills? Perplexed, Richard could not come up with an answer. We suggested that he explore new activities outside work, but that seemed impractical to him, and he left the office feeling as down as ever.

The answer came to Richard the next evening. He and his wife Helen had been thinking of purchasing a cooperative apartment for investment. If they could buy an apartment where Richard could be an active part of the board, then he could find an entire range of interesting work activities *away* from his job. A few days later, the Michaelses began apartment hunting in earnest. Some months later, they owned a lovely apartment, and Richard and his wife quickly became members of the co-op board. Six months later, Richard was elected president of the board, whose members recognized his talents and genuine wish to be involved.

Although still entrapped at work, Richard, guaranteed a good salary until retirement, felt he had a new lease on life. "It was a boon," he said. "I could negotiate with contractors and tradesmen, get estimates, make recommendations to the board, manage money, do all the things I used to do at work. But right in my own backyard! And Helen is going to be our next treasurer, so we'll have plenty to do."

This case illustrates important aspects of emotional entrapment and how it can be effectively handled. One solution to entrapment is to quit the situation entirely. But sometimes a job change or transfer is unrealistic and therefore not a viable way out of such a bind. In these cases, something else must be done. Richard Michaels took an important route to minimize his own obvious entrapment. He discovered a new activity and revitalized his life. This discovery was more than simply finding a new hobby; his involvement on the co-op board minimized his frustration with work, reducing the job's role in his life. For Richard, finding another source of gratification in his life was an effective and realistic solution to his entrapment. With this new-found activity, his chest pains subsided almost completely.

Finding new, meaningful sources of pleasure is an important way to cut down on a major entrapment and involves, in part, a reassessment of your priorities and goals as described in step 1. Steps 1 and 2 (reordering priorities and decreasing emotional entrapment) really go hand in hand. Opening yourself to new pleasures can help you find a new dimension in your life and decrease your sense of entrapment.

Many patients redirect themselves to new priorities and pleasures only *after* they have had an encounter with illness and the possibility of death. However, you need not develop heart disease nor must you survive a heart attack to reorient your perception of stultifying emotional traps that have enslaved you.

Many people live their lives in an emotional "neutral gear," waiting for some as-yet-unknown pleasure magically to materialize. They hunger for some unidentified, unattainable goal. Such striving for poorly defined goals leads to smoldering feelings of discontent and despair. These emotions activate a primitive physical response which can eventually destroy their hearts and their lives.

Discovering new and challenging ways to spend time rather than yearning for a vaguely happy future requires harnessing your emotional energies in a positive way. It means making more efforts to derive pleasure on a day-to-day basis. The benefits are twofold; you can actually feel that you have something worthwhile in your life, and your body is spared the physical effects of all the bad feelings.

Trapping—and Beating—Invisible Entrapment

Entrapment also occurs in a variety of everyday situations, at work and in our personal lives. Less dramatic than, say, a tumultuous marriage, these less obvious life traps often go unnoticed. We call this *invisible entrapment*.

Relatively minor, everyday traps can be a potent source of frustration, resentment, and other negative feelings that can wear down your heart. One of the most dangerous aspects of invisible entrapment is that it can produce continuous stress. Many of these traps can occur together over months or years, and the effects on your morale and on your heart accumulate.

The following case is an example of invisible entrapment taken from our practices.

> Charles Benson had been an angina patient for three years. He decreased many ongoing stresses in his life, lost weight, exercised regularly, and was doing quite well. One situation, however, still "made his blood boil" and brought on chest pains.
>
> Charles had been friendly with George Harper since their college days, when they were both single. George had recently divorced and remarried. The Bensons remained friendly with George after the divorce, and now that he was remarried, they frequently spent time with George Harper and his new wife Sue.
>
> Unfortunately, Sue was hostile toward anyone from George's "former" life. Each evening spent as a foursome exposed Charles to Sue's barbs, provocative comments, and mean-spirited unpleasantries. Whenever the Bensons returned home from an evening with the Harpers, Charles experienced pressing chest pains that he feared could escalate into a heart attack.
>
> Charles and his wife discussed this situation several times and decided that he could not afford such tension; it was exacting a toll from his health. But Charles felt entrapped. He didn't want to lose George's friendship, but he couldn't tolerate his friend's wife.
>
> After some thought, Charles decided to change subtly his relationship with George Harper. He began inviting George to

lunch. After a few months, a pleasant lunchtime pattern was established, and the two old friends would enjoy themselves as they had in earlier days. In a sense, the relationship reverted back to its original form. This ongoing contact eliminated the need for them to get together with their wives. With this new arrangement, no one's feelings were hurt, nothing unpleasant was said, and Charles didn't have to tolerate George's wife. The Bensons and the Harpers got together as couples only once a year, and Charles and his wife (and Sue, no doubt) considered this a more acceptable alternative.

So ended a small, potent form of invisible entrapment in Charles Benson's life. He rarely experienced angina pains after that.

Charles Benson's invisible entrapment shares certain characteristics with Richard Michaels' obvious entrapment. In each situation the victim felt snared and could not see his way out of the bind. Each situation had a no-win quality. And each man's heart paid the price.

However, there are important differences between these two forms of entrapment. Richard's obvious entrapment was a bind he could not control; he made no contributions to the trap. Charles's invisible entrapment, however, depended on his own wish not to insult his friend. Charles's own feelings played a part in his entrapment. Invisible entrapment usually depends on the unknowing participation of the victim.

Invisible entrapment taps the following feelings, and then the trap is set:

1. You feel obligated, as though you owe something to another person.
2. You fear you will be disliked or unloved.
3. You don't want to seem selfish, hurt someone's feelings, or deprive or disappoint someone.

These feelings boil down to two basic human fears:

- Fear of losing the affection or love of someone you think you need
- Fear of feeling bad about yourself (guilt)

Each victim contributes these two basic fears to his or her own invisible entrapment. The following are examples of everyday emotional binds that can make you feel invisibly entrapped. You can easily recognize the two fears that help snare the victim and form an effective entrapment.

1. For years, you've been spending simply awful Sundays with your in-laws. They're overbearing and critical, and the evenings always end in a series of arguments. You hate going, but altering this well-entrenched routine will make your husband and in-laws feel hurt and rejected, making *you* the bad guy. Reluctantly, you find yourself preparing for yet another Sunday hassle. You get heartburn and a headache every time you go.

2. It's been a rough week and you have the beginnings of a cold. You really don't feel up to it, but you can tell from your wife's signals that she wants to make love. If you don't show enough interest, she'll feel hurt and rejected. You decide to just go ahead. After all, you pay a smaller emotional price if you make love, even if tonight lovemaking seems like an obligation.

3. This is the fifth time that your wife has invited the Johnsons to a dinner party. They haven't reciprocated in over a year, and frankly, you find it annoying that the relationship is so one-sided. Your can't blame your wife. After all, since the Johnsons know the other guests, if they weren't invited, they would find out about the party anyway. They would feel hurt, maybe even resentful.

You don't need resentment to build up, especially since you and Al Johnson work together. It's a bind, and you can do nothing but grin and bear it. Still, it would be nice if the Johnsons were more sensitive or at least demonstrated a sense of fair play. You try to shrug it off, but you feel every muscle in your body tightening up as you open the door to the Johnsons.

4. It's the thousandth time a check has bounced. Your husband never keeps the balance and sometimes forgets to enter the amount of the last check. And then he can't remember how much it was. How come you have to organize everything having to do with money and budgeting? And you have to arrange all the details for vacations too. These pounding headaches are getting worse. You just *know* it's your blood pressure.

5. It's been going on for years now; every time you go out with the Smiths, you pick them up and do the driving. Either something is wrong with their car or something pops up—you always end up driving. It's inconvenient and unfair. Do you look like a chauffeur?

6. Your brother, sister, cousin—everyone, it seems—needs help. And they always come to you—to cash a check, to give a small loan, to give tax advice or help with their returns. Or they borrow books (which they don't return) or tools, whatever. It never stops. You know these constant demands make your blood boil, and your blood pressure shoots sky-high.

How to Decrease Invisible Entrapment

Minimizing invisible entrapment is not complicated and doesn't require that you revolutionize your life. It does mean rethinking and reordering certain priorities about yourself. Above all, you must commit yourself to decreasing the small, but potent, sources of entrapment and stress in your life. Here's how:

1. Scan your work and social life to determine sources of invisible entrapment. Include relationships with your spouse, friends, relatives, and coworkers. You will be surprised to see how many minor traps there are in your life.

2. Decide which ones you no longer wish to tolerate.

3. Recognize that your fear of losing someone and of feeling guilty do not necessarily reflect reality. The truth is, very few people will hate you for acting more self-interested—if you do it the right way.

4. Lessen entrapment without shouting "no!" Think about *alternatives to the situation* you wish to change. Do what Charles Benson did; find an acceptable way to continue the relationship on different, more tolerable terms. Examine the six examples, and figure out compromise solutions for each. Most of them require better communication with your spouse and a compromise that will be the least likely to offend anyone.

5. Once you've found your own traps, think of workable compromise solutions, just as you did for our examples. There are more than you think. Remember, the solution doesn't have to be radical.

6. Most invisible entrapment situations can be changed without ending the relationship. In rare instances the only way to minimize entrapment is to make such a drastic move. Usually that relationship is really quite dispensable once you decide that *your feelings* and *your heart* count for more than preserving a guilt-ridden or one-sided relationship.

7. Even if you cannot minimize the power of a particular situation to entrap you, just realizing you are trapped and seeing clearly the situation will make you feel much better. Sometimes simply defining a problem can limit its power over you.

8. Above all, deciding to minimize intolerable emotional traps (both obvious and invisible) requires taking a stand against a variety of impositions and stresses that can wear away at your heart. Take charge of your life!

Step 3: Modifying Type A Behavior

By now you have probably taken an emotional inventory of yourself and know what you must do to live a longer and healthier life. Step 3 is very important if you recognize type A behaviors in your life. You must modify these behaviors and tone down your fight-or-flight responses in daily life. You will save your heart from a great deal of wear and tear.

If you are like most people who rate high in type A behavior patterns, you may be thinking: "But haven't these personality traits helped me get where I am? Haven't they been important to my success? Aren't these personality characteristics inborn? If they aren't, isn't it true that they're part of me, and I can't change them? After all, wasn't my personality formed by the time I was six years old?"

First, type A behaviors are not personality traits. Type A behavior has been erroneously labeled a "personality" or "character type," as though it were some character disorder or psychiatric diagnosis. It is not. The concept of type A describes certain coronary-prone *behaviors*, nothing more. Some personality types may exhibit more type A behaviors than others, but these behaviors are seen in many people with varying makeups and character traits. If this world had only two kinds of people—type As and type Bs, say—it would be a dull and dispirited place. Clearly, to describe the totality of human nature, character, and purpose as either type A or type B is a gross oversimplification.

Since we're not talking about changing the very fabric of your nature or individuality, we must define *modifying type A behavior*. The key word here is *behavior*. We urge you to consider modifying certain learned behaviors: certain ways of moving, walking, talking, and interacting that you have *learned* and that have become part of the way you do things. You can modify these behaviors to reduce their frequency or intensity, or you can "unlearn" and eliminate them. Drs. Friedman and Rosenman called this kind of behavioral change "reengineering."

You may argue that type A behavior is responsible for your present success—unquestionably, some type A qualities do contribute to success. However, they also contribute to your having had a heart attack or your angina pectoris!

In truth, achievement-oriented and reasonably competitive elements in your personality (along with other things such as imagination, brains, daring, and energy) are responsible for your success, not type A behavior. As a matter of fact, type A behavior is often seen in people who are not particularly successful. You may have succeeded because of some type A behavior, say, getting things done quickly but well, or you may do well in spite of certain type A behaviors which can be abrasive and off-putting to other people. Remember, these behavioral patterns are evident in people of different personality types; some are successful, and some are not.

Equally important, hard-core type A patterns often limit and interfere with your enjoyment of success. Since you are always rushing to acquire new possessions, earnings, or accomplishments, you cannot appreciate what you already have.

In short, if you rate high in type A behaviors, you pay an enormous price for any success that you may have, finding it difficult to do more than scurry about acquiring additional things at the expense of beauty and enjoyment. Type A behavior is no bargain!

How do we know that type A behavior can be changed? In 1984, a federally financed study of more than 800 men recovered from heart attacks demonstrated that counseling to reduce type A behavior cut in half the chances of a second heart attack.

The study, conducted by Dr. Meyer Friedman, used psychological guidance to curb the main characteristics of type A behavior: time urgency, competitiveness, and free-floating hostility. Men who went through the program were able to modify many type A behaviors and reduce the risk of having another heart attack. Type A patterns were reduced in 80 percent of patients given type A counseling: the counseling consisted of 44 group sessions over a three-year period. If three years seems a long time, remember that the patients had severe heart disease and most had deeply ingrained type A patterns.

The sessions were conducted by specially trained group leaders. Patients were given descriptions of type A behavior and then shown videotapes of their own activities. Recognizing their explosive speech patterns and tendency to interrupt others, some could not bear to watch themselves. The patients were given drills that encouraged reducing the pressure to rush through things and to be constantly aware of time. They practiced being pleasant to other people, trying to appreciate beauty and find time for activities that enriched their senses.

The results of this study were dramatic. Counseled to relax and learn different behaviors, men stricken by heart attacks had fewer second attacks and lived longer. These findings are significant not only for people who have had heart attacks, but also for those who are not patients.

How can these findings benefit you? Certainly, few readers who rate high in type A behavior patterns are about to enroll in an expensive three-year course involving group sessions and videotaping. Moreover, to the best of our knowledge, no such program is now available to the general public. However, the most important parts of the program offered by Friedman and Rosenman in their book *Type A Behavior and Your Heart* (Fawcett Crest Publications, 1974) are outlined in this step. For a complete review, we recommend their book. The following pages borrow from them, modifying their suggestions to fit our Heartplan strategy for improved health and good living.

Before You Begin

Changing something so complex as behavior may seem like a tall order, but it may be much easier than you think. If you've decided to follow step 1 of Heartplan to set new priorities and realistic goals, you've already taken enormous strides toward modifying crucial aspects of your thinking, your feelings, and your way of doing things! Recall Dr. Striver from step 1. He made no conscious attempt to modify any of his type A behaviors, yet, in his rethinking and remodeling of certain parts of his life, these behaviors began to change.

A genuine commitment to reorienting your priorities and goals means that heart-damaging behaviors may already be falling by the wayside. In a real way, you've made a commitment to life and to improving the *way* you live, and thus changing type A behavior quirks may not be so hard. After all, motivation is nearly everything.

Only six group therapy sessions with recovered heart attack patients resulted in dramatic improvements in a study done by Dr. Richard Rahe. Patients in those groups were able to change their overwork habits (a Sisyphus trait) and reduce their sense of time urgency (type A behavior). The large-scale study by Friedman merely confirms Dr. Rahe's observations. Perhaps the intense counseling reported in the new studies isn't always necessary; with the proper awareness and motivation, people may be able to change certain behaviors in far fewer sessions.

Probably you've been totally unaware of your self-damaging ways of thinking, feeling, and behaving. Take personal stock of yourself, and you will discover a new-found awareness of the need to change certain areas in your life. Awareness of a problem is often 90 percent of the solution.

Changing behaviors doesn't mean revamping everything or making a totally new you. Rather, the change focuses on the one or two areas you need to modify and on doing something about them. A sense of time urgency and free-floating hostility are the two features of type A behavior most easily modified. They both compromise your heart and your ability to enjoy life.

Hurry Sickness

Although Friedman and Rosenman suggest drills to counteract what they call "hurry sickness," the suggestions that follow are not really drills. They are an outline to use to decrease your sense of time urgency, the need to rush everything in your life. Some are easy to do; others are more difficult.

1. Keep in mind your constant rushing from one place or thing to another. Be aware that you make too many appointments or take on too many projects each day or week. Stay aware that you do things too fast, as though the sole object of your activities is merely to finish them. Try to eliminate rushing in even the most ordinary ways. Walk, talk, and eat more slowly. Pace yourself when you work, when you walk down a street, when you talk. Ask yourself, "Why am I rushing? Is this worth dying for?" Chew your food slowly; savor the flavors. Make yourself stay at the table even if you've finished eating before everyone else. These restraints can be difficult at first, because they remind you how quickly you do most things. Awareness (even if it's painful at first) is most of the battle.

2. Learn to loaf. Put your mind and body into neutral gear; this probably contrasts with the way you've done things for years. Try loafing for 5 minutes in the morning and 5 minutes in the afternoon. Expand your loafing time to a half hour and then a full hour each day, either during the day or in the evening.

While loafing, rethink the day's pleasant events, *not* the hassles and stresses. Dwell on the most pleasant thing that happened to you all day. If nothing pleasant happened, think back on the week and find something; make it the core of a daydream.

3. Remind yourself that a job or task need not be accomplished in record time to be done well. As a matter of fact, slowing down will probably help you get much more done, and you'll probably get it done better. Look for pleasure in the doing of things, not only in looking back on a task completed. Virtually any activity has an inherent pleasure; you need not look very hard.

4. Set up a system of self-reward. Whenever you know you haven't rushed through a day or if you know you've been prudent or circumspect in a situation, arrange to give yourself something of value. This pertains to business meetings (where you don't interrupt and where you bite your lip), tasks around the house, driving in traffic, going leisurely from one appointment to another, and other newly hurry-free aspects of your life.

Make slowing down pleasurable by rewarding yourself for it, even if you don't now particularly like the slowed-down pace. You are using *positive reinforcement* by rewarding yourself for positive, healthy behaviors and not rewarding or punishing for negative, unhealthy ones. The way that type A behaviors drain away life's pleasures and the effect such behavior has on your heart are punishment enough. The reward can be anything—dinner at a favorite restaurant (we'll show you how to eat at any restaurant and still eat healthfully) or a bottle of your favorite wine. You decide.

5. Force yourself to browse, shop, bargain hunt, or window shop for a definite period each day. Whether you stroll through a bookstore, record shop, arcade, pet store, gallery, museum, flower shop, or any other place with wares on exhibition, you will benefit. Such activity demands that you take time out and slow down, and soon browsing becomes its own reward. Certain stores will attract because of dimly recalled preferences (for instance, a pet store), and long-forgotten memories and dim flickerings of childhood interests will surge back into your mind, if only for brief moments or faded flashes. These memories will intensify over time, and you will find yourself on a journey of rediscovery. The pleasures of these moments will prime you for others, and you will become more willing to live amidst these pleasures of the moment. Your life and heart will improve.

6. Force yourself to leave your wristwatch at home. You will find this painful at first, but it will have an impact on you in many ways. You will discover how many times each day you take meaningless glances at your watch, as though time is about to catch up with you and do you in. Practice a little "timelessness."

7. Remind yourself every day that many things will go undone in your life and that the most worthwhile things are never truly finished—love, commitment, family, friendships, and the beauty of the world. These realizations help you to reorder your life's priorities, and they go hand-in-hand with reducing your time urgency.

Lessening Combative Hostility

If you are easily aroused to hostility or simmer with combative readiness, you must strive to eliminate this mind-set as much as possible. Nothing can excite your entire fight-or-flight system quite as effectively as hostility and combat. We again borrowed from Friedman and Rosenman in forming our strategy for lessening combative hostility:

1. Smile at strangers in the street, on elevators, and in other places. This may seem silly or even hypocritical, but it can pay

enormous dividends. Smiling is contagious; when people see you smile at them, they do so in return. You will be amazed at how warm many people are willing to be; they will reciprocate a friendly greeting with pleasure. This is a form of positive reinforcement that amply rewards your efforts.

2. Try doing something nice and unpredictable for your spouse; buy a small gift, say, go out to dinner on a night when it would be unusual, or suggest a three-day weekend at a resort. Whatever you choose will generate good feelings and will be a source of positive reinforcement.

3. Play a game and plan to lose. See if you can take it. Practice losing, and make a joke out of it. Try to enjoy the other person's triumph. There's nothing humiliating in losing. A variation of this is to admit to someone that you're wrong, even if you aren't. Enjoy the surprise on the other person's face.

4. Avoid other angry, combative, and competitive people who rate high in type A characteristics. The last thing you need is to feed each other's fires. Remind yourself that your readiness to respond to challenges has already taken its toll on your heart; work at ignoring challenges large and small. Learn to laugh at yourself and at those who challenge you in various ways. Rise above them.

Changing detrimental behaviors is not very difficult. You *can* do it once you:

- Reorder your life's priorities and set new goals.
- Make a genuine commitment to live your life as fully and richly as possible.
- Identify heart-damaging behaviors and decide which ones must be changed.
- Open yourself to positive reinforcement from yourself, other people, and, most important, your spouse. Start now!

Step 4: Reducing Both Large and Small Stresses

You woke up this morning feeling edgy about things at the office. You're not getting along with the new administrative assistant.

To make matters worse, you had another argument with your wife. Rushing to work, you got stuck in traffic, and the car began acting up again. When you take the car in (if you can find the time), you'll take the 7:15 for a day or so, but that train always runs late.

These ordinary stresses and hassles can fill anyone's day. Some seem trivial; others more important. Some may be the warning signals of momentous upheavals in your life. They can take an enormous toll from your emotional and physical well-being. Before we discuss reducing your stress load, let's divide stress into three types: major life changes, chronic or ongoing stress, and minor irritants.

Major life changes usually alter the fabric of your life. They include such events as the death of a loved one, divorce, marriage, retirement—any important change in your work or living arrangements. These events, whether happy or tragic, call for an adaptive response when they occur.

Chronic or ongoing stresses are usually less evident than a major life change, although they can lead to such a change. For example, a troubled marriage can eventually lead to a separation or divorce. Ongoing stresses include trouble with the boss, dissatisfaction with your work, financial troubles, and a variety of other frictions and problems.

Minor irritants are the stuff of everyday life—losing your wallet, getting stuck in traffic, a spat with your husband or wife (sometimes not minor), rushing to make a deadline, any of a long list of seemingly trivial but irritating stresses from which no human being is immune.

Different people have different thresholds for stress, and something that bothers you may not trouble someone else. However, stress is part of everyone's life, and it requires adaptive coping responses. How you deal with stress is especially important if you are a cardiac patient, since your heart is affected by stresses large and small.

The following pages outline various ways to deal with the three types of stress. Remember, it is not stress itself that causes physical and emotional trouble; rather, how you *respond* to stress makes the difference between health and illness. As helpful as our strategies for dealing with stress may be, there is no way completely to avoid turmoil in your life. A life without stress is not a life at all.

Dealing with Major Life Changes

Try to avoid too many major life changes within any given year. Of course, some events are beyond your control—the death of a loved one or friend, a merger or bankruptcy at work, a job layoff, and so on. But you can control the timing of some life changes. For instance, if you have recently married or just had a baby, consider putting off other important changes such as purchasing a new home or making a job transfer (these last two events frequently occur in a "package"). Many people cope with this combination of changes, but they are stressful all the same.

As a rule, it's better to pace major events so that you don't feel deluged by overwhelming changes. Although there are exceptions, it's best to take one step at a time.

Dealing with Chronic or Ongoing Stress

We see many cases in which conflict between husband and wife (or between parent and child) triggers angina attacks. This conflict is a chronic stress whose source must be discovered and dealt with so that your heart doesn't pay the price.

When a family relationship is a source of ongoing conflict and strife, psychological counseling for all involved family members can be very helpful. The goal here is not to bring about deep personality changes. Rather, counseling can help family members (especially a heart patient) find different ways of coping with their conflicts to reduce friction in the household.

Chronic stress situations may occur at work. Try to minimize them by changing the particular aspect that bothers you. A transfer or shift to another location, if possible, or a frank talk with your colleague or boss to work out differences, are attempts to defuse the ongoing stresses in your life.

For some people, even minor hassles are sources of chronic stress, because they habitually overreact. Increased awareness of such a tendency can bring about changes in your attitudes and behaviors. The key is to develop insight about situations that cause daily strife and thus have potentially bad effects on your heart. Don't underestimate the power of your own awareness.

David Brewster was a 50-year-old man being treated for angina. He quickly named an ongoing stress factor in his life: his need to respond to any small provocation as though it were a major challenge. Even minor annoyances could shred his composure, causing him to blow up. In short, he'd never learned to walk away from a fight.

Increasingly aware of this vulnerability, David and his wife told us about the following situation: The couple got into a taxi and asked the driver to take them downtown. The driver refused, saying he was heading toward his garage; he would only take an uptown fare. David's immediate impulse was to start steaming and argue with the man, who technically was obligated to drive them to their destination.

Instead, David turned to his wife and suggested that they get another taxi. "We'll let this guy get another fare," he said. With that, the couple left the taxi. "I can't tell you how good it made me feel," David said. "Arguing would have shot my blood pressure up. Getting out of the taxi was my way of telling this guy that he wasn't important in my life. Not at all. It made me a winner."

David had converted a no-win situation into one where he felt he had won. To argue would have been bad for his blood pressure and his heart. To allow himself to be bullied would have been bad for his self-esteem. He did neither. Instead, he defused the situation and laughed it off. David was learning to walk away.

People who are hot reactors in specific situations can use relaxation techniques in these settings. Research has shown that these techniques—meditation, self-hypnosis, and deep muscle relaxation—can reduce the fight-or-flight response during periods of emotional arousal. The techniques also can produce a sustained calming effect beyond specific stressful situations. Your blood pressure and heart rate will benefit from use of these techniques.

Dealing with Minor Irritants

Life's little hassles can sometimes appear to outweigh major misfortunes as a source of trouble to your health. Early studies of stress focused almost entirely on major life changes, but it now seems clear that less traumatic situations often contribute to an overall stressed feeling. Recent research has shown that people who face an intolerable number of minor irritants have poorer mental and physical health than do people who actually deal with a major life crisis!

Sometimes, a major life change sets into motion a variety of irritations that extend the impact of the event. For instance, losing your job puts you under stress because of the emotional impact of finding yourself unemployed, and you must deal with a shaken self-image. On another level, the job loss disrupts the established patterns of your life. You now worry about paying bills; you have long spans of idle time; you stand on the unemployment line and arrange job interviews. The job loss has swept you into a series of daily hassles.

Many of life's small stresses are unavoidable, no matter where you live or work—the country, the city, or a suburb. Most everyday hassles have certain things in common; they involve senseless waiting under crowded conditions, unexpected delays or mistakes, and an unsettled feeling that you no longer completely control your fate. You can feel helpless, tense, angry, and overwhelmed. There are so many common irritations in life that we often fail to recognize them as stressful situations.

Although you cannot make life hassle-free, you can take the stress out of certain situations. The following pages present common trouble spots and some practical strategies for reducing the frequency and impact of these petty annoyances.

AT THE BANK

Banks can be maddening places. Here are some ways to keep hassles to a minimum:

- Avoid banking during lunch hours, on days when Social Security checks arrive, and on days when quarterly interest is updated.
- Use automatic teller machines whenever possible. Rarely crowded, they are reliable and hassle-free.
- If a hospital or large corporation is located near your bank, find out when payday falls. Avoid banking on those days.
- Find a bank that stays open in the evening and on Saturday. Not all banking must be done on weekdays between 9:00 and 3:00.
- When you enter a bank, if you see long lines, leave and return in a few hours or the next day. Frittering your lunch

hour away on a bank line can upset you. If you must stay, try people watching. It can be interesting.
- Plan ahead. Establish when you will need money in your checking account so that you can avoid a last-minute rush and an imperative visit that can put you on a bank line.

AT THE SUPERMARKET

Some people are fond of supermarkets; for others, they are an exercise in stress and irritation. Long delays at the checkout are annoying. Your heart and blood pressure may pay the price. Here are some tips for reducing supermarket-related stress:

- Use a supermarket with plenty of checkouts. Many supermarkets are converting to electronic checkers, which are more efficient.
- Find a supermarket that stays open twenty-four hours a day and shop when shoppers are scarce. Beware of Friday evenings—supermarkets are often crowded just before weekends.
- Avoid major shops just before big holidays such as Christmas and Thanksgiving. A supermarket is a madhouse at these times.
- A patient of ours and his wife cut down on supermarket delays in the following way: Their shopping list rarely contains more than 20 items. They divide the list in half, take two shopping carts, and get their items. Then, one behind the other, they speed through the express lane (you are allowed 10 items per person), avoiding the congestion of the regular lanes.

COMMUTING

Commuting is a daily source of tension for millions of Americans. It can be the bane of your existence if you face an arduous trip each morning and evening. Try some of these tips:

- Avoid driving if you can. If a good commuter railroad is available, use it. Your trip can be a special part of your day if you approach it correctly. Make it "private" time. You can do paperwork without telephone interruptions (but try to avoid being a Sisyphus). You can read, knit, think, or fantasize about your wildest dreams. If you are the sociable type, find others like yourself. Some commuters board the same car and take the same seats each day, making the trip a social situation. Some commuters play cards.

- Buy commuter tickets in advance. This will avoid a hassle at the station, especially if you're running a bit late.
- If you drive, find a route that is less heavily trafficked, even if it is a little longer. It'll spare your arteries and your heart.
- Try staggering your work schedule. Can you come to work earlier or later? You may be able to avoid the inbound and outgoing rushes each day.
- If you get stuck in a traffic jam, try to be philosophical. Occupy your mind with a pleasant thought or a fantasy. Listen to a provocative talk show on the radio. Getting steamed won't make the traffic move faster.

DOCTOR APPOINTMENTS

Although many doctors try to work on schedule, they often fall behind, and you can wait for hours in a doctor's office. To avoid sky-high blood pressure, follow these suggestions:

- Treat your own time as a valuable commodity. When calling for an appointment, ask if the doctor "runs late" or if appointments are kept at the specified time. Plan accordingly.
- For a routine visit, request an appointment that makes you the first scheduled patient.
- If your appointment is in the middle of the day, call an hour or two ahead and ask if the doctor is running on time. If not, how far behind schedule are things going? Plan accordingly.
- Don't schedule nonemergency dental appointments during late August or early September. School children get dental checkups then, and you'll wait for hours.

VACATIONS

Following a few simple rules will undoubtedly make for a much less stressful vacation. Here they are:

- Make reservations early. Remember, vacations are for enjoyment, not hassles. One sure-fire way to feel hassled is to begin or end a vacation waiting at a crowded airport when flights are backed up. If waiting annoys you, don't schedule departures or return flights on summer weekends or during peak holiday periods.
- When going abroad for a summer vacation, get your passport months before you plan to leave. Applying for one during the summer guarantees you long waits and hot tempers.

SERVICE AND TRADES WORKERS

Television repairers, electricians, and other tradespeople can be a source of hassles if you don't take the right steps:

- Schedule service visits for first thing in the morning so you won't be trapped at home all day.
- If the delivery or service cannot be scheduled for early morning, plan activities to fill the day so you don't gnash your teeth while you wait. Plan to work at home or use the time productively.
- Confirm all appointments a day ahead so that you're reasonably certain that you won't be waiting for nothing.

GENERAL STRATEGIES FOR DEALING WITH MINOR HASSLES

We have touched on some specific everyday hassles; obviously life offers many more. The following are some strategies to apply to your particular minor stress:

- Learn how you cope with hassles best. Does it help to discuss the situation with a friend? If so, make time to do so. Do you find it helps to cry or laugh? Laughing can be particularly good medicine. Whichever response—laughing or crying—makes you feel better is probably the best one for you. Think about how you cope best and then follow through. You will learn to cope more effectively with minor stresses.
- The best coping style is to avoid the stress, but sometimes you cannot. Then you must try to minimize the impact of

the stress. If you must deal with a hassle, make a contract with yourself, that is, plan to reward yourself after the situation fades. Give yourself something special (a good bottle of wine, dinner at your favorite restaurant). Visualizing this reward even as you handle the stressful situation will let you feel that something positive is coming out of your troubles.

- If you find that a few minor hassles are getting you worked up, look inside yourself for something deeper. "Talk" to yourself: "Is something *else* really bothering me?" This internal scanning can be very helpful.

    Mel Roberts suddenly found noise around the house unbearable. The noise came from the usual things: the kids playing the television too loudly or running around. He began snapping and having minor flare-ups. Scanning why this was happening, he realized the true source of his annoyance: The office was especially hectic and his secretary was out sick. Mel was deluged with work, and his office worries made ordinary minor household hassles loom larger than they really were. He was scapegoating his children.

- When dealing with minor stresses, don't let your body get involved. In other words, don't let your temper flare up such that your entire fight-or-flight system gets thrown into high gear. Be careful, though—smothering feelings can also cause stress. Instead, try to look for the funny side of the situation; defuse the annoyance. For instance, you called the roofer to estimate replacing the shingles on a small section of roof. She quoted the ludicrous price of $5000. You can laugh at this absurdity, because the job isn't worth nearly that much and you know it. Obviously the roofer is booked full and doesn't want a small job unless she gets paid a small fortune. You'll find another roofer who is reasonable.

- Remember, some stress—large or small—is inevitable. Although a little foresight and planning can cut down on some common irritations, you will still face occasional trouble spots. How well you cope will determine how much they bother you. A sense of humor can lighten the impact

of these hassles, and keeping the larger life issues in their proper perspective will help you to avoid getting charged up and damaging your health.
- There are two rules for maintaining your perspective when dealing with minor daily stresses: (1) Don't sweat the small stuff. (2) It's all small stuff!

Step 5: Eating for Health and Pleasure

Let's face it, dieting is a bore. Happily, this step is *not* a diet; it is about eating well and eating right. The following are basic principles for healthy eating:

1. Eating is one of life's pleasures. Don't forgo or diminish that pleasure.
2. Continue eating many of the foods you now enjoy; you just need to modify them somewhat.
3. Don't become obsessive about every calorie or each milligram of sodium, cholesterol, or fat. Rather, you can change what you eat without feeling deprived and without feeling that your entire life revolves around dieting.
4. Continue dining at restaurants and at friends' homes without worrying that the foods you eat are bad for you.

You already know that cholesterol, fats, and hypertension are major contributors to the "sludge" that can form in your coronary arteries and lead to heart disease. You also know that to modify the risk factors of too much cholesterol, fat, and sodium, you must eat less of these substances. Food will still taste good—changing the way you eat doesn't mean deprivation!

The suggestions on the following pages are based on guidelines established by the U.S. Department of Health, Education and Welfare, the U.S. Senate Select Committee on Nutrition and Human Needs, and the American Heart Association. We have made many modifications in these guidelines and have added some of our own.

Although these suggestions were established for patients with heart disease, they can also be used by people who wish to avoid heart trouble. If you have a genetic condition resulting in very high levels of blood fats, you may need some special modifications. Diabetics can follow this diet, but they must carefully avoid simple sugars—those not found naturally in fruits or juices.

Suggestions for Eating for Health and Pleasure

1. Attempt to reach and maintain your ideal weight. If you need to lose weight, do so gradually while developing a new consciousness about food that will last you a lifetime. Avoid crash or fad diets that mean losing large amounts of weight in a short time or that severely restrict the variety of foods they allow (for instance, "the grapefruit diet"). Ideal weight is most easily maintained by balancing your caloric intake with physical activity.

2. Eat a variety of foods to make meals interesting. Include items that contain protein, carbohydrates, and some fats. Complex carbohydrates (potatoes, pasta, rice, and certain vegetables, cereals, and breads) should be the major source of calories. Intake of saturated fats and cholesterol should be as low as possible.

3. One major way that people gain weight is by eating large portions. Cut down the size of your portions, especially meats. Eat more vegetables, fruits, legumes, and unrefined carbohydrates such as potatoes, rice, pasta, and whole-grain breads.

4. Make routine meals very low in calories, fat, and cholesterol. Do what we call "calorie banking." Save up for special meals by minimizing your intake of fats and cholesterol during ordinary meals. For instance, on weekday mornings, you don't need a large breakfast with eggs, butter, and the like. Have bread or cereal and coffee or tea. Don't use cream or sugar; if you use good coffee, you don't need to add anything to it. You can buy exotic beans and grind them yourself. Eat a European breakfast: bread or rolls with a small amount of jelly along with your coffee.

Save up for that special Sunday breakfast, brunch, or dinner with friends when you may want to splurge. Splurging means *some* fat, but don't gorge yourself. An occasional meal that contains fat and extra calories isn't going to do you in, especially if you've banked calories beforehand. Remember, the overall, steady intake of too much fat, cholesterol, and calories does the most harm, not the occasional mild indiscretion.

Avoid liquids that contain calories. Drink seltzer, club soda, water, diet sodas (sodiumfree), tea or coffee with no sugar or cream.

Calories contained in liquids can really add up; for instance, each large glass of fruit juice adds 100 calories, and enough glasses can be transformed into pounds of gained weight.

5. Severely limit your intake of foods high in cholesterol and saturated fats. Eat no more than three egg yolks a week. Don't overlook hidden sources of egg such as cake mixes and certain breads. Avoid most red meat; organ meats such as liver and kidney; bacon; sausage; corned beef; pastrami; most luncheon meats such as salami, bologna, liverwurst; frankfurters; and fatty ham. When you do eat these things, limit your portion to 4 ounces or less. (This is a small portion. Most Americans eat 10 to 16 ounces of meat per portion.) Limit your intake of butter, cream, whole milk, sour cream, ice cream, whipped cream, and sweet cream. Rich, processed cheeses (usually soft in consistency) are best avoided. Cheese spreads and American cheese are particularly bad. Don't eat any cream cheese—it's loaded with fat! Use low-fat goat cheese products and skim milk cheeses. Other low-fat cheeses (between 20 and 45 percent fat) such as Jarlsberg, mozzarella, Parmesan, ricotta, and Romano are okay in limited amounts. Peanut butter, nuts, and olives should be limited.

6. Milk and dairy products that are skimmed or low in fat are fine. You can choose between milks that are skimmed and have virtually no fat or those that contain $1/2$ percent or 1 percent milk fat instead of the usual 3 percent milk fat found in whole milk. Once you get used to these lower-fat milks, whole milk will taste unpleasantly creamy to you. Yogurt made from skim milk is delicious and healthful.

7. Use small amounts of cooking oils. Polyunsaturated oils are preferable. Such oils are liquid at room temperature, including sunflower seed oil, safflower oil, corn oil, soybean oil, cottonseed oil, and sesame oil. Olive oil is monosaturated, that is, it is more easily turned into saturated fats once it's in your bloodstream, so use olive oil in limited amounts. (Recent evidence, however, points out that monosaturated olive oil may be as good as the polyunsaturated oils.) Avoid saturated oils such as coconut and palm oil; they are basic building blocks for saturated fats and cholesterol in your body. Remember, all oils are pure fat, which means they're loaded with calories.

Avoid all solid fats, hardened oils, lard, or vegetable shortenings used in commercial baking. They're loaded with saturated fats. Also, watch out for cream substitutes and whipped cream toppings—they are filled with coconut oil, palm oil, and other saturated fats.

Beware of one other thing. Nowadays, advertisers are well aware that many consumers avoid or minimize cholesterol. Because products are advertised as having "no cholesterol" does not mean that they're good for your heart. They can be loaded in polysaturated fats! A recent advertisement said, "Olive oil has no cholesterol!"—a statement that is technically true. However, olive oil is still pure fat and should not be liberally used.

8. When cooking with oils, especially when sautéing in a pan, use a nonstick frying pan to minimize or even eliminate the use of oil. The water released by vegetables makes a good sauté medium, along with a little white wine. You can even add a little water to increase the liquid content in the pan.

9. Margarines that come in tubs are preferable to those that come in sticks. They contain more liquid polyunsaturated oil (which is the first ingredient listed on the label). When reading labels, beware of any ingredient listed as "vegetable oil": if the exact oil isn't specified, the chances are high that it is coconut or palm oil; both are polysaturated. Remember, *any* margarine—no matter which kind of oil is used—is fat and loaded with calories.

10. Avoid commercially baked products which use vegetable shortenings that are high in hydrogenated or saturated oils. And avoid chocolate; it's cocoa and fat. Also, commercial candy bars often contain coconut or palm oil, which, again, are not good for you.

11. When preparing red meat, make certain the cut is as lean as possible. Then trim off all visible fat. Cooking over a grill, spit, or barbecue are the best methods, since they allow fat to drip away. Broiling and baking are fine too. Avoid frying foods; allowing the food to sit in its own fat maximizes the amount of fat and cholesterol. Above all, avoid commercially fried foods of any kind; they're loaded with fat.

12. Try cutting down your meat consumption. We've been programmed to think of meat as being *the* food for a main course, and for many people a meal without a large portion of meat seems incomplete. Meat need not be the centerpiece of a meal: It is only one of many components making up a dining experience. You don't need a 12- or 16-ounce slab of beef on your plate to eat a "real" meal.

The Italians have mastered the art of eating better than we Americans have. An Italian meal may start with a light antipasto and a small portion of pasta and be followed by a small piece of grilled meat, veal, or chicken with vegetables. The salad comes next, followed by coffee and dessert. Thus the meal comprises a series of smaller servings over a longer time, in contrast with the American style of piling everything onto the plate at one time. Try the Italian method of serving courses.

Eat more carbohydrates. Try eliminating any kind of meat on one or even two or three days each week! Be creative; think of ways to replace meat. Eat rice, pasta, potatoes, and other complex carbohydrates. Limit meat to a small amount contained in the sauce used on pasta or rice.

Another way to cut down on meat is to eat liberal amounts of salads and vegetables. Fresh, properly cooked vegetables are delicious, and here the key is learning to get *fresh* produce (shopping for the best and freshest can be great fun). You must also learn the best method for cooking produce. A first course of salad (with an appropriate dressing made with polyunsaturated or monosaturated vegetable oil) can be very satisfying and filling. More salad and a variety of vegetables can accompany the main course.

13. What foods are best for you? All complex carbohydrates such as pasta, good whole-grain breads, rice, and grain cereals are fine, as are fish, poultry (chicken or turkey, without skins), shellfish (up to a limit), mollusks, veal, center-cut loin of pork, cottage cheese, fruits, skim milk, yogurt, and fruits and vegetables. Fresh vegetables can be a delight, and getting them fresh entails eating different vegetables according to the season. Frozen and canned lose a lot in the translation.

Starting a strict, low-cholesterol, low-fat diet is tough. We usually recommend a rigid diet for the first two months, with almost no cheating. It takes two months to find foods you like and to learn to cook in innovative ways. The diet may be unpleasant at first, and you won't like everything, but your tastes will change. You will learn where to buy good ingredients and how to cook them in interesting ways—use a variety of spices and herbs liberally. Remember, the way you eat is a habit that takes time to change.

Freshness counts—especially with vegetables and fish! Years ago, one of the authors (Dr. Copen) introduced his children to fish—they hated it. Then he learned where and when to get fish very fresh—the day the supplier came back from *his* supplier. Suddenly the kids loved fish!

14. Be imaginative. You can have great fun thinking up ways to prepare and cook foods to taste delicious and be low in cholesterol and saturated fats. Regard this as a new and exciting change in your life. Devote time and effort to it—become a food aficionado. Discovering new tastes can be exciting. Try asparagus, artichokes, and snow peas. Visit an oriental market, and you'll find incredible vegetable tastes and consistencies.

New treats await you. Freshly made mozzarella cheese is heavenly, as are some of the low-fat goat cheeses. Incredibly delicious breads are waiting to be discovered. Nearly every city or town has an ethnic bakery. Eat freshly baked breads instead of the bland packaged varieties. As for gravies, make them more interesting by adding herbs. Refrigerate gravy until the fat forms on the top, and then skim it off.

15. Shellfish is fine, although some tends to be a little high in cholesterol. Shellfish is so expensive that most people eat only small quantities of it, especially in restaurants. Shrimp should be eaten in small quantities; the little shrimp has a lot of cholesterol. Scallops, crab, and lobster are good, but don't dunk the pieces into drawn butter. Mollusks—oysters, mussels, and clams—are fine too, but watch out for the rich, creamy sauces often served with them. A fish called pollock has the taste and consistency of crabmeat (some call it "mock crab") but is lower in cholesterol. Dipped in cocktail sauce, it's a dead ringer for Alaskan king crab, but less expensive.

16. Substitute ingredients to eliminate high-fat and cholesterol-loaded items from your daily fare. To evaluate foods and recipes for fat, assess the *quantity* of fat. A small amount is no problem. You don't have to count calories fanatically to slim down and stay at a reasonable weight. Nobody gains weight by eating normal amounts of foods that are low in fat and cholesterol, because the concentrated calories are removed.

Try out new recipes from any cookbook; even those with the richest recipes can be used *if* you substitute ingredients. This can be fun and delicious.

The following is a family recipe that we will present and then modify, to lower fat content.

Paupiettes (Veal Rolls in Sauce)
(serves four)

4 veal scallops (cutlets)	1 stalk celery, finely chopped
4 slices of swiss cheese	1 carrot, finely chopped
1 clove garlic, pressed	1 onion, finely chopped
1/2 teaspoon marjoram	1/2 cup dry white wine
1/2 teaspoon rosemary	1/2 cup beef broth
Salt and pepper to taste	1/2 teaspoon thyme
5 tablespoons butter	1 bay leaf
1 tablespoon olive oil	1 tablespoon all-purpose flour

Pound scallops thin. Combine garlic, marjoram, rosemary, salt, and pepper. Spread evenly over scallops. Cover with a piece of cheese. Roll scallops as for a jelly roll. Tie with string.

Melt 4 tablespoons of the butter with oil in frying pan. Add celery, carrot, and onion. Cook until golden, stirring frequently. Stir in wine and broth; add thyme, bay leaf, salt, and pepper. Mix well. Pour into a baking dish. Place veal rolls in sauce. Cover. Bake in a preheated 350°F oven, one shelf below center, for 1 hour and 30 minutes. Remove casserole from oven; lift out veal rolls to serving dish. Keep warm.

Remove bay leaf from sauce. Pour sauce into food processor; puree.

Melt 1 tablespoon of butter in saucepan; stir in flour to make a roux (smooth paste). Pour in sauce, stirring constantly; bring to a boil. Reduce heat; simmer until sauce thickens. Remove string from veal. Pour sauce over veal. Serve with potatoes or rice.

Now for the modification. We will transform this recipe into a delicious low-cholesterol and low-fat experience:

3 carrots, finely chopped	4 parsley stalks
1 extra large sweet onion, finely chopped	1 tablespoon polyunsaturated vegetable oil
3 stalks celery, finely chopped	4 chicken breasts, boned, skinned, and butterflied

$1/2$ cup clear saltfree chicken broth
$3/4$ cup dry white wine
$1/2$ teaspoon thyme, twice
1 bay leaf

Pepper to taste
1 medium clove garlic, finely minced
$1/2$ teaspoon marjoram
$1/2$ teaspoon rosemary

Utensils
1 large nonstick skillet
Mortar and pestle
Baking dish with cover

Preheat oven to 350°F. Melt 1 tablespoon oil in nonstick skillet. Add carrot, onion, and celery; cook until golden, stirring frequently. From this mixture, set aside 2 tablespoons of sautéed vegetables for chicken filling. To the ingredients remaining in the skillet, add the wine, chicken broth, bay leaf, $1/2$ teaspoon of thyme, parsley stalks, and a dash of freshly ground black pepper. Stir to mix well. Set aside.

Pound chicken breasts between two pieces of waxed paper. Trim any fat. In a mortar, combine the 2 tablespoons of sautéed vegetables, garlic, marjoram, rosemary, and $1/2$ teaspoon thyme. Work with the pestle until all ingredients are mixed to a coarse paste. Place a spoonful of the paste on one-half of each butterflied chicken breast, and then fold the other half of the breast over the mixture.

Pour the reserved vegetable, wine, and broth mixture into a baking dish. Place the chicken paupiettes in the sauce. Cover. Bake one shelf below the center of the oven for approximately 45 minutes or until done. Remove the casserole from the oven; place chicken rolls on a serving dish. Keep warm. Remove bay leaf and parsley stalks from sauce; pour sauce into blender or processor. Puree.

Pour vegetable mixture puree over chicken. Garnish with finely chopped parsley.

Serve with boiled new potatoes or rice.

The following changes transformed the recipe into a low-cholesterol, low-fat dish:

- Substitute chicken for veal.
- Omit butter and olive oil (use scant amount of vegetable oil with specially treated skillet).
- Omit cheese and substitute with vegetable filling for chicken center.
- Omit flour.

These changes reduced the dish's sodium content:

- Omit salt.
- Omit beef broth; substitute saltfree chicken broth.
- Add celery for extra flavor.

We personally attest that this dish, made in the low-cholesterol, low-fat style, is delicious.

17. When shopping, familiarize yourself with labels. Remember, product ingredients are listed in descending order for quantity. If a label lists salt as third or fourth, the product is probably loaded with salt. Although you don't need to read every word in every label, you should be able to make sense out of any label. Remember that a product whose label lists "vegetable oil" or "partially hydrogenated vegetable oil" contains saturated fat and should be avoided.

18. Never add salt to your food. Many people are so accustomed to salt that they consider it "the flavor" of many foods, much to the impoverishment of their palates. Once you've cut down on salt, you'll be surprised how the brine-laden taste of heavily salted food becomes somewhat offensive. It masks the subtler tastes that can make eating a delight. Learn to use spices and herbs; there are dozens that you can use to make food taste great.

Many people cook vegetables in water, which depletes them of their natural flavors. Instead, steam vegetables to preserve flavor and consistency. Then, salt won't be needed to add taste.

19. Avoid obviously salted foods such as potato chips, salted pretzels, and corn chips. Use garlic and celery powders, not the flavored salts. Of course, it's best to use fresh ingredients whenever you can, but the powders can add flavor.

STEP 5: EATING FOR HEALTH AND PLEASURE

The following foods are very high in salt (sodium) and are best avoided, especially if your blood pressure is high:

garlic salt   *pretzels (salted)*
onion salt   *soy sauce*
pickles and pickle relishes   *steak sauces*
potato chips (salted) *Worcestershire sauce*

Beware of sodium in foods that contain preservatives such as sodium citrate, sodium benzoate, and sodium tartrate.

20. Healthy, tasty food requires time and effort to obtain and to prepare properly. Such care is never taken in fast-food establishments, and the flavor of nearly all "junk" food is based on an excess of salt, sugar, or burnt fat! These taste enhancers can make the most poorly prepared, worst-quality ingredients taste acceptable. Fast-food establishments make an enormous profit by selling a high volume of low-quality food that is quick and easy to prepare. We consumers pay a price—the sludge that collects in our arteries!

There are no shortcuts to tasty, nutritious, low-fat meals. If you want to eat well and enjoy healthy, tasty food, you must devote effort to shopping and preparation. It's worth it!

21. For dessert, fresh fruits are best. They change with the season, perhaps offering tastes you've never had before. Find the best produce stores you can; get to know them and learn more about fruits and vegetables.

Desserts can be diet wreckers, but they don't have to be. For starters, it can be fun to discover dozens of delicious, low-calorie, low-fat desserts. Gelatin, angel food cake, sherbet, and ice milk are just a few; use your imagination to come up with many more.

A recent addition to the fat watcher's list of desserts is Tofutti, a cholesterol-free but caloric substance made from bean curd. It has the taste and consistency of ice cream and comes in many flavors. Tofutti is now sold in bulk packages and in individual servings.

The previous pages set forth guidelines to help you begin and maintain healthful eating habits. You must do a little work, but the effort is worthwhile. The key is to find good sources of fresh produce, breads, pastas, and spices. Then take the time to prepare and cook them so that they're delicious—time and commitment are essential. You will eat healthfully while still anticipating delightful meals. Lean cuisine need not mean dull food!

Dining at Friends' Homes

One of the most unpleasant experiences you can have is to invite a friend to dinner at your home, only to discover that he or she is "on a diet" and cannot partake of the feast you've prepared. You wouldn't want that happening to you, nor should you do it to others.

If you are a cardiac patient, good friends will often inquire about any special diet preparations or restrictions. Depending on your relationship, you may or may not feel free to make a request. You must be the judge.

Let's say that you are given no choices. You can enjoy yourself without making a big deal about your new style of dining. If you've wisely calorie-banked (having known about the dinner for at least one week) don't hesitate to partake of your host's generosity. If red meat is served, you can enjoy a slice or two and eat heartily of vegetables, potatoes, breads, salads, and whatever else is served. Remember, it's your *overall, steady consumption of fat and cholesterol* that counts most, not the occasional indulgence.

You don't have to be a fanatic. Avoid telling friends and relatives that you're on "this diet" that sets you apart from the rest of the world. The diet may seem strange to them, and furthermore, can make you feel as if you are depriving yourself. Eat with the others, keeping in mind that even while having a sumptuous meal at someone else's home, you can use discretion.

Dining at Restaurants

Many people assume that eating healthfully means forgoing dining at most of their favorite restaurants. This simply is not true. For many people, dining out is a great pleasure, and there is no reason that you cannot continue eating at your favorite restaurants. Some modifications are in order, but they don't preclude enjoying yourself.

Use common sense. Don't expect restaurant chefs to prepare complicated, cholesterol-free dishes that aren't on the menu. Most restaurants will gladly broil or poach a piece of fish in water (with some wine and lemon juice) and serve it with vegetables and potatoes. All fish is fine as long as it's not fried. Chicken can be broiled or baked and enlivened with a variety of herbs and spices or a good barbecue sauce. You need not feel deprived. As at home, rely on salads, vegetables, and complex carbohydrates (potatoes, pastas, and rice) to round out any meal.

We include here a simple guide to cholesterol-free dining at various ethnic restaurants.

AMERICAN STEAK HOUSES

Except for an occasional indulgence in red meat, steak houses are best avoided. When you do go, share one portion of steak among two or three people, and eat more salad, potato, and bread. Otherwise, stick to broiled chicken or poached or broiled fish, which many good steak houses do very well. However, since it can be depressing to eat such fare while everyone else tears into juicy red meat, avoidance is the best policy.

GERMAN AND EASTERN EUROPEAN RESTAURANTS

German and Eastern European cuisines are very heavy and depend to a great extent on creamy, rich sauces for their character. Watching your fat intake while dining at such restaurants is quite difficult.

ITALIAN RESTAURANTS

Italian restaurants provide a wealth of wonderful dishes, but beware of Northern Italian cuisine, which often uses creamy white sauces. Southern Italian cooking is more likely to offer an assortment of delectable, low-fat possibilities. Here, too, watch out for pastas stuffed with fatty meats and whole-milk cheeses. Also, some tomato sauces can contain *prosciutto* (Italian ham) or *pancetta* (cured bacon), so inquire before ordering.

Italian pastas and seafoods are great and can be fatfree, if you know what to choose. Order pastas with marinara sauce, tomato sauce, red or white clam or mussel sauce, garlic and oil, or oil and vegetables (so long as it isn't boosted with cream). Any pasta will do. When ordering fish, stick to those called *posillipo*, *Livornese*, *marechiare*, and *brodetto*. Any *zuppa di pesce* (fish soup) is likely to be delicious and low in fat. Other winners are cold seafood salads (usually drizzled with a little olive oil), green salads, vegetables, and roasted peppers.

CHINESE RESTAURANTS

Chinese restaurants present problems for the prudent diner or for anyone trying to limit salt intake. Unfortunately, Chinese cuisine depends on heavy doses of soy sauce and peanut oil for flavoring, resulting in salty, oily food. Eggs can be hidden in fried rice and noodle dishes, and bits of ham are often tossed into various dishes for added flavor.

You're best bet is to stick with vegetable dishes, provided that they aren't oil-soaked (which can happen with stir-fried creations). You can enjoy steamed fish with a variety of vegetables, bean curd, scallops, and chicken dishes (provided they aren't fried or too oily). Ask the waiter to have the chef go light on the oil (usually peanut oil, which is quite saturated), although in our experience these instructions often go unheeded.

JAPANESE RESTAURANTS

Much to our delight, Japanese restaurants are proliferating rapidly in many areas of the United States. *Sushi* and *sashimi* may turn you off if you think of them as raw fish, but once you've tasted them, they are wonderful. Just don't use soy sauce. One glance at any Japanese menu will clearly indicate many fish and chicken dishes that are cooked in their own broth or broiled. They are usually served with a tempting variety of oriental and domestic vegetables, steamed and spiced exotically. Again, watch the soy and salt intake.

MEXICAN, TEX-MEX, AND SPANISH RESTAURANTS

Authentic Mexican cuisine is very hard to find in the United States. What we've learned to call "Mexican" is really Tex-Mex, a U.S. variation of Mexican cooking. Authentic Mexican fare presents a wide variety of fish, chicken, and other meat cooked in various ways, some very low in fats, others high.

Tex-Mex restaurants present a problem because many of their dishes are fried and oil-soaked. In addition, this cuisine tends to be quite salty, so if you're watching your blood pressure, it may not be for you. Stick with tacos and tostadas stuffed with shredded chicken or refried beans. Avoid the heavy, oil-soaked chiles *rellenos* and other fried Tex-Mex items.

Some Mexican restaurants have a section of menu reserved for Spanish dishes. Spanish cuisine offers many dishes that are low in fat and a delight to the palate: *mariscadas* (shellfish) in green sauce; *zarzuella*, a Spanish version of the Italian *zuppa di pesce*; and nonseafood dishes such as *arroz con pollo* (chicken with rice).

FRENCH RESTAURANTS

Although French cuisine presents many possibilities, limiting your intake of cholesterol and saturated fats in a French restaurant will require some adroit choices. As most people know, French cooking uses plenty of cream and butter in sauces, and you must search French menus carefully for low-fat dishes.

Most French restaurants offer a lovely variety of raw vegetables for hors d'oeuvres, and they are certainly safe. Also, salads and mussels prepared *marinière* (mainly with wine and broth) are usually among the hors d'oeuvres. Dishes labelled *Provençal* (sauteed in olive oil with garlic and herbs), various chicken stews (such as *coq au vin*), and other fish and chicken dishes are fine. A good rule of thumb is that French restaurants poach fish beautifully, but order the cream-and-butter sauces *on the side*. A light dab of sauce on each mouthful provides wondrous taste and limits your intake of calories and fats.

About Desserts

The dessert cart in many restaurants (especially French and Italian) can be a mouth-watering temptation for even the most resolute soul. For safety's sake, stick with sherbets, fruits, and other low-fat (and less exciting) offerings. If you can't hold back, try splitting a dessert with one or two other people. After all, many desserts are so rich that just a taste will satisfy.

A great way to avoid desserts is to order an espresso as dessert and ask the waiter to add some anisette. This delightful concoction will fill up that last bit of you begging for more. With a drink such as this, who can feel deprived?

About Alcohol

Meals at home or in restaurants may seem more exciting with wine or another alcoholic beverage. This is fine, as long as you drink moderately—one or two cocktails per day or two glasses of wine with a meal.

Eating Out Is Good for You

In the past, eating prudently while dining out was difficult. Today, more restaurants are accommodating the public's awareness of the need for low-fat, delicious food. Restaurants are offering more seafood, poultry, fresh vegetables, salads, and fruits along with interesting breads. More menu items are steamed, grilled, broiled, and poached instead of deep-fried. Sauces tend to be lighter and more sparingly used.

Some local chapters of the American Heart Association (AHA) publish a dining guide that details strategies for healthful eating. Some AHA chapters recommend specific restaurants that will accommodate diners with special needs. Call your chapter to find out if this service is provided. Also, many restaurants (from the most elegant to fast-food concerns) now have a special menu with low-fat, low-cholesterol dishes, including the Sheraton, Fairmont, Hilton, Stouffer, Westin, Marriott, and Four Seasons hotel chains.

Most airlines also offer low-calorie, low-cholesterol, and low-sodium fare for their health-conscious passengers. As public awareness increases, more restaurants and hotels will provide a variety of healthful foods to make your dining life pleasurable. Dining out *is* good for you psychologically, and, if you eat right, it's good for your heart as well!

The Heartplan Program for Day-to-Day Great Eating

The following pages provide a 28-day program for eating according to our Heartplan principles. One of the authors (Dr. Rubinstein) followed these daily menus for 28 days and then remained on a modified Heartplan program.

These suggested menus are guidelines for how easy it is to enjoy healthful food and reap the benefits of the Heartplan program. The menus contain a variety of interesting foods. The meals are simple and easy to prepare; all ingredients are readily available in grocery stores and require no complicated shopping ventures.

These menus will appeal to all family members, whether or not they are Heartplan followers. The meals are balanced each day for cholesterol, sodium, calories, fiber, and protein. A very high premium is placed on taste! Remember, portions of meat should not exceed 4 to 5 ounces; while vegetables, complex carbohydrates, and fruits can be eaten in liberal quantities.

To maximize benefits from the Heartplan program, plan a week's worth of menus at a time. Take into account dining out or special occassions during the week (you will see how Dr. Rubinstein did this in the following pages). Remember to allow for calorie and cholesterol banking.

The lunches are specially designed to be easily prepared to eat at home, to take to work, or, in most instances, to order in a restaurant. This allows for a maximum of flexibility.

A cornerstone of any eating program is allowing for sufficient quantity of food with plenty of variety and taste so that you don't feel deprived. Using our Heartplan menus not only will be good for you, it may actually spice up your dining experiences! Follow this menu guide for 28 days, or prepare your own using the easy principles we've outlined. Certain Heartplan dishes are marked by an asterik (*), which indicates that the easy-to-follow recipe is given at the end of this step.

Before we present the menu plan, let's look at Dr. Rubinstein's cardiac profile before he began the Heartplan program.

Age: 43
Height: 5'10"
Weight: 188 lbs.
Blood pressure (average, at rest): 130/88

Average resting pulse: 68/min.
Cholesterol: 205
Triglycerides: 85
HDL as compared to total cholesterol: 26.8% (below-average cardiac risk)

SUNDAY, DAY 1

Sunday Brunch
Fresh fruit cup
Heartplan French Toast*
Beverage (coffee, tea, club soda, low-calorie soft drink, or mineral water)

Afternoon Pick-Me-Up
Cup of vegetable soup
One slice of whole-grain bread (no butter or margarine)

Dinner
Tomato and mozzarella slices with basil vinaigrette
Baked herbed chicken breast (remove skin before eating)
French-style green beans tossed with water chestnuts
One glass of wine
Slice of angel cake
Beverage

MONDAY, DAY 2

Breakfast
Grapefruit juice
Bowl of high-fiber cereal with low-fat milk
Beverage

Lunch
Tuna salad on whole-grain bread (water-packed tuna, drained and tossed with low-fat mayonnaise)
Beverage

Dinner
Tossed green salad
Pasta *primavera* (using a tomato-based sauce with fresh seasonal vegetables)
Two glasses of wine
Two oatmeal cookies (baked without hydrogenated oils; available at any health-food store)
Beverage

TUESDAY, DAY 3

Breakfast
Piece of seasonal melon
Toasted roll with low-sugar jelly
Beverage

Lunch
Cup of vegetable soup
Tossed salad
Beverage

Dinner

Tomato, cucumber, and sweet onion salad
Broiled salmon steak
Heartplan wild rice with mushrooms*
One bottle of light beer
Baked apple
Beverage

WEDNESDAY, DAY 4 (no meat or fish)

Breakfast

Medium banana
Cottage cheese on cinnamon toast
Beverage

Lunch

Lettuce and tomato sandwich on whole-grain bread
Fresh fruit cup
Beverage

Dinner

Cold asparagus vinaigrette
Rigatoni with Heartplan marinara sauce*
Two glasses of wine
Low-sugar sherbet
Beverage

THURSDAY, DAY 5

Breakfast

Small glass of grapefruit juice
Bowl of high-fiber cereal with low-fat milk
Beverage

Lunch

Breast-of-turkey sandwich on whole-grain bread (low-fat mayonnaise or other low-fat dressing only)
Beverage

Dinner

Tossed green salad
Heartplan vegetarian chili*
Corn muffin

One bottle of light beer
Piece of fresh fruit
Beverage

FRIDAY, DAY 6

Breakfast

Half of a grapefruit
Toasted whole-wheat English muffin with low-sugar jelly
Beverage

Lunch

Spinach and mushroom salad (no bacon; only whites of hard-boiled egg)
One slice of whole-grain bread
Beverage

Dinner

Heartplan coleslaw*
Heartplan crunchy baked fish*
Steamed broccoli
Baked potato (add a dollop of low-fat plain yogurt with fresh chives instead of butter, mayonnaise, or sour cream)
Two glasses of wine
Piece of fruit
Beverage

SATURDAY, DAY 7

Breakfast

Small fresh-fruit cup
Toasted bagel with low-fat cottage cheese
Beverage

Lunch

Piece of fresh fruit (calorie banking—dinner will be at a restaurant)
Beverage

Dinner at an Italian Restaurant

Mussels *posillipo*
Tossed salad
Broiled veal chop
Two glasses of wine

Bread (no butter)
Fruit tart
Espresso with anisette

SUNDAY, DAY 8 (no meat or fish)

Brunch

Half of a grapefruit
Heartplan omelet*
One slice of whole-grain toast
Beverage

Snack

Fresh-fruit cup with low-fat plain yogurt
Beverage

Dinner

Tossed green salad
Heartplan stuffed peppers*
One bottle of light beer
One slice of angel cake
Beverage

MONDAY, DAY 9

Breakfast

Small glass of grapefruit juice
Toasted bagel with low-sugar jelly
Beverage

Lunch

Sardine sandwich with lettuce and tomato on whole-grain bread
Beverage

Dinner

Tossed green salad
Heartplan chicken marsala*
Heartplan wild rice*
Two glasses of wine
Piece of fruit
Beverage

TUESDAY, DAY 10

Breakfast
Piece of melon
Bowl of high-fiber cereal with low-fat milk
Beverage

Lunch
Cup of Heartplan gazpacho*
Two slices of whole-grain bread
Beverage

Dinner
Sliced tomatoes and sweet onions
Flounder fillet steamed in white wine in foil packet
Heartplan spicy string beans*
Two glasses of wine
Beverage
Oatmeal cookie

WEDNESDAY, DAY 11 (no meat or fish)

Breakfast
Small glass of grapefruit juice
Two slices of whole-grain bread with low-fat cottage cheese
Beverage

Lunch
Fresh-fruit salad with one scoop of low-calorie sherbet
Beverage

Dinner
Tossed green salad
Vegetable stew on rice
Two glasses of wine
Beverage
Slice of angel cake

THURSDAY, DAY 12

Breakfast
Half of a grapefruit

Toasted whole-wheat English muffin with low-sugar jelly
Beverage
Lunch
Cup of vegetable soup
Tossed green salad
Beverage
Dinner
Pickled green beans
Broiled halibut steak
Steamed new potatoes with dill
Two glasses of wine
Beverage
Scoop of vanilla-flavored Toffuti

FRIDAY, DAY 13

Breakfast
Piece of melon
Cinamon toast
Beverage
Lunch
Sliced breast of turkey with lettuce and tomato
One slice of whole-grain bread
Beverage
Dinner
Tossed green salad
Linguine with white clam sauce
Two glasses of wine
Fresh-fruit cup
Beverage

SATURDAY, DAY 14

Breakfast
Glass of grapefruit juice
Bowl of high-fiber cereal with low-fat milk
Beverage
Lunch
Cup of tomato soup

Step 5: Eating for Health and Pleasure

One slice of whole-grain bread
Beverage

Dinner

Dinner was eaten at friends' house; the friends don't follow the Heartplan program, and no special request was made. Dishes available were:

Appetizers
Crudités with cheese dip
Assorted cheese tray
Shrimp cocktail with sauce
Stuffed eggs

Entree
Tossed salad with Roquefort dressing
Roast prime ribs of beef
Yorkshire pudding
Broccoli with hollandaise sauce
Assorted rolls
Wine

Dessert
Fruit tarts and mini-eclairs
Coffee and tea
Cordials

Dr. Rubeinstein's selections were:

Appetizers
Crudités (plain, or very light on the dip)
Shrimp with cocktail sauce (6)
No cheese tray, no stuffed eggs

Dinner
Tossed green salad (very light on the dressing)
One slice of prime rib of beef
No Yorkshire pudding
Broccoli (without hollandaise sauce)
Two rolls (no butter)
Two glasses of wine

Dessert
Fruit tart
Coffee
After-dinner cordial
No mini-eclair

124 STEP 5: EATING FOR HEALTH AND PLEASURE

SUNDAY, DAY 15

Breakfast
Half of a grapefruit
Two slices of whole-grain bread with low-sugar jelly
Beverage

Lunch
Tuna salad on whole-grain bread (tuna packed in water, served with low-fat mayonnaise)
Beverage

Dinner
Tossed green salad
Paillard of chicken breast
Baby carrots and fresh peas
Steamed new potatoes with tarragon
One glass of wine
Beverage
Fresh-fruit cup

MONDAY, DAY 16 (no meat or fish)

Breakfast
Bowl of high-fiber cereal with sliced banana and low-fat milk
Beverage

Lunch
Lettuce and tomato sandwich
Beverage
Two oatmeal cookies

Dinner
Cucumber salad
Heartplan Indian vegetable casserole*
Scented rice*
One bottle of light beer
Beverage
Slice of chilled papaya with lemon

TUESDAY, DAY 17

Breakfast
Piece of melon

Cinnamon toast
Beverage
Lunch
Cup of tomato-based fish chowder
One slice of whole-grain bread
Beverage
Dinner
Tossed green salad
Heartplan German-style potato salad*
Cold poached chicken breast with mustard sauce
Two glasses of wine
Beverage
Slice of angel cake

WEDNESDAY, DAY 18

Breakfast
Small glass of grapefruit juice
Toasted whole-wheat English muffin with low-fat cottage cheese
Beverage
Lunch
Breast-of-turkey sandwich (with low-fat mayonnaise) on whole-grain bread
Beverage
Dinner
Sliced tomato, cucumber, and onion salad
Heartplan marinara sauce on pasta*
Garlic bread sticks (dietetic—purchase at a health food store)
Two glasses of wine
Scoop of ice milk

THURSDAY, DAY 19

Breakfast
Half of a grapefruit
Toasted roll with low-sugar jelly
Beverage
Lunch
Spinach salad (no bacon, only the whites of the hard-boiled egg)

Beverage
Two oatmeal cookies

Dinner

Tossed green salad
Chicken cutlet parmigiano (use low-fat mozzarella and Heartplan marinara sauce)
Steamed zucchini with oregano
Two glasses of wine
Beverage
Piece of fresh fruit

WEDNESDAY, DAY 20

Breakfast

Bowl of high-fiber cereal with sliced banana and low-fat milk
Beverage

Lunch

Fresh-fruit salad with scoop of low-fat cottage cheese
Small plain bran muffin
Beverage

Dinner

Tossed green salad
Fish stew with vegetables
One bottle of light beer
Sourdough bread
Beverage
Low-sugar sherbet

SATURDAY, DAY 21

Breakfast

Small glass of grapefruit juice
Heartplan omelet*
Beverage

Lunch

Cup of vegetable soup
One slice of whole-grain bread
Beverage

Dinner (at home with four visitors)
Heartplan eggplant spread on high-fiber crackers*
Mock crab with cocktail sauce
Crudités with fresh-herb dip (use low-fat plain yogurt)
Tossed green salad
Heartplan chicken paupiettes on a bed of wild rice* (see recipe above)
Assorted breads
Two glasses of wine
One large slice of lemon chiffon pie
Beverage
One after-dinner cordial

SUNDAY, DAY 22

Brunch
Piece of melon
Bagel with low-fat cottage cheese and smoked salmon (2 thinly sliced pieces)
Sliced ripe tomatoes and sweet onion
Beverage

Snack
Piece of fruit

Dinner
Tossed green salad
Roast cornish hen
Baked sweet potato
Steamed asparagus
One bottle of light beer
Beverage

MONDAY, DAY 23 (no meat or fish)

Breakfast
Small glass of grapefruit juice
Toasted whole-grain English muffin with low-sugar jelly
Beverage

Lunch
Cup of tomato soup

Two slices of whole-grain bread
Beverage
Piece of fruit

Dinner

Cucumber salad
Stuffed cabbage (filled with brown rice, onions, and mushrooms)
Stewed tomatoes
One bottle of light beer
Beverage
Scoop of Tofutti

TUESDAY, DAY 24

Breakfast

Half of a grapefruit
High-fiber cereal with sliced banana and low-fat milk
Beverage

Lunch

Lettuce-and-tomato sandwich on whole-grain bread
Beverage
Two oatmeal cookies

Dinner

Tossed green salad
Baked red snapper
Steamed new potatoes with dill
Sautéed spinach with water chestnuts
Two glasses of wine
Beverage

WEDNESDAY, DAY 25

Breakfast

Piece of melon
Two slices of whole-grain toast with low-sugar jelly
Beverage

Lunch

Sardine sandwich on whole-grain bread
Beverage

Dinner

Tossed green salad
Stuffed pasta shells with tomato sauce (fill shells with low-fat ricotta cheese)
Two glasses of wine
Beverage
Slice of angel cake

THURSDAY, DAY 26

Breakfast

Small glass of grapefruit juice
Cinnamon toast
Beverage

Lunch

Breast-of-turkey sandwich on whole-grain bread
Beverage

Dinner

Heartplan coleslaw*
Small center-cut loin pork chop, broiled
Low-sugar applesauce
Steamed green beans with caraway seeds
Beverage

FRIDAY, DAY 27

Breakfast

Half of a grapefruit
Bowl of high-fiber cereal
Beverage

Lunch

Fresh-fruit salad with one scoop of low-fat cottage cheese
Beverage

Dinner

Tossed green salad
Broiled scallops with ginger
Bran rice with snow peas
One bottle of light beer

Beverage
Scoop of ice milk

SATURDAY, DAY 28

Breakfast
Fresh-fruit cup
Heartplan French toast*
Beverage

Lunch
Cup of vegetable soup
One slice of whole-grain bread
Beverage

Dinner (at a Chinese Restaurant)
Chicken with watercress (request very little oil)
Sautéed broccoli with garlic sauce (request very little oil)
Steamed rice
One bottle of light beer
Beverage
Pineapple chunks

Preparing Special Heartplan Dishes

The following is a simple guide to preparing the special Heartplan foods mentioned in the preceding menu plans. These dishes—through use of a few simple substitutions—are low in fat and cholesterol and very high on taste and nutritional value! Most dinner recipes can be prepared easily in less than one hour.

Heartplan French Toast
(serves two)

2 thick-cut slices of bread (at least 1-day old)
2 egg whites
2 tablespoons low-fat milk
Sprinkle of cinnamon and nutmeg
$1/4$ teaspoon orange extract

Combine all ingredients except bread and beat lightly. Dip bread into mixture, coating well. Lightly oil a nonstick skillet; when skillet is hot, fry bread on both sides until golden. Serve with fresh berries, low-sugar jelly, or a trace of maple syrup.

Heartplan Omelet
(serves one)

Prepare your favorite omelet mixture, but substitute 2 egg whites and 1 whole egg in place of the usual 2 to 3 eggs. Remember to use low-fat milk and fry in a lightly oiled nonstick skillet or omelet pan. It's delicious!

Heartplan Gazpacho

Use your favorite gazpacho recipe, but omit oil and salt and increase the amount of celery. This produces a saltlike taste without increasing sodium content. You'll be amazed at how delicious this mixture is, and it uses no oil!

Heartplan Wild Rice with Mushrooms

Wild rice is generally available in supermarkets and health food stores. Do not use a package of premixed rice and mushrooms; these all contain hydrogenated oils and plenty of salt.

Cook rice according to directions given; omit butter or oil and salt. A salt-free chicken broth can be substituted for water to heighten flavor. While rice is cooking, sauté fresh sliced mushrooms in a little oil and white wine. Season with freshly ground pepper. Combine cooked rice with mushrooms and serve.

Heartplan Vegetarian Chili
(serves four)

Assemble your favorite vegetables, but be sure to include:

1 large onion, thinly diced
1 clove garlic, finely minced
2 stalks celery, chopped
1 carrot, thinly diced
1 red pepper, chopped
2 cups peeled whole tomatoes
1 can (10 1/2 ounces) low-salt tomato soup
1 teaspoon sweet paprika
chili powder (to taste)
1/8 teaspoon cayenne pepper
1 can (16 ounces) red kidney beans with low-salt liquid
1 1/2 tablespoons vegetable oil

Heat oil in a cooking kettle or large skillet. Sauté the onion, garlic, celery, carrot, and red pepper until soft. Add the tomatoes, soup, and spices, mixing well. Simmer for 5 minutes. Cover. Simmer over low heat for 1 hour, stirring occasionally. Add kidney beans with their liquid. Heat through and serve. Absolutely wonderful!

Heartplan Coleslaw

Use your favorite coleslaw recipe, but substitute low-fat mayonnaise for whole-egg mayonnaise, and cut back on the amount added. You'll never know the difference!

Heartplan German-style Potato Salad

Use any German-style potato salad with these changes: decrease the mayonnaise, and use only low-fat mayonnaise; do not use bacon or the yolks of hard-cooked eggs; add thinly diced red and green pepper, radishes, and scallions or sweet onions for color and flavor. It's great!

Heartplan Stuffed Peppers

Prepare pepper shells according to your usual method for baking, or refer to any standard recipe.

Stuff peppers with a mixture of cooked rice, sautéed onion and green pepper, diced and peeled tomato. Add your favorite seasonings (remember to limit salt). Top with bread crumbs and a sprinkle of Parmesan cheese, and then dot with margarine.

Bake in a 350°F oven for 30 minutes.

Heartplan Spicy Green Beans

(serves four)

1 tablespoon oil
1 small onion, diced
1 clove garlic, finely minced
1 tablespoon oregano
1/2 teaspoon thyme

1 bay leaf
1 cup peeled tomatoes
1 cup low-salt tomato juice
1 pound string beans

Heat 1 tablespoon oil in a nonstick skillet. Sauté 1 small onion, diced, and 1 clove garlic, finely minced, until soft. Do not brown mixture. Add 1 tablespoon oregano, $1/2$ teaspoon thyme, and 1 bay leaf. Sauté for 5 minutes.

Add 1 cup peeled tomatoes and 1 cup low-salt tomato juice, bring mixture to a boil. Add 1 pound French-style string beans, cover, lower heat, and cook until beans are cooked through but not soft. Add fresh-ground pepper and a drop or two of squeezed lemon before serving.

Heartplan Indian Vegetable Casserole

(serves four)

1 medium onion, diced
2 stalks celery, diced
2 carrots, diced
2 medium potatoes, peeled and diced
1 red pepper, diced
1 green pepper, diced
1 chicken bouillon cube
2 to 3 tablespoons curry powder (depending on strength and preference)
1 teaspoon paprika
$1/4$ teaspoon chili powder (use less if powder is very hot)
$3/4$ cup low-fat milk
2 cups peeled tomatoes
$1/2$ package frozen peas, thawed
$1/4$ cup raisins
1 zucchini, sliced
1 small head of cauliflower, broken into florets

Sauté onion, celery, carrots, pepper, and potatoes until the potatoes are almost cooked through. Do not allow the other vegetables to brown. Sprinkle the spices over the mixture and cook for 5 minutes.

Add the bouillon cube and the milk. Stir constantly until the mixture boils. Lower heat and add the tomatoes. Simmer gently for 15 to 20 minutes.

Add the peas, raisins, zucchini, and cauliflower. Cook until the vegetables are *al dente* (do not overcook). Serve with scented rice.

Heartplan Scented Rice

Prepare a package of long-grain rice according to the directions, but remember to omit butter, margarine, oil, and salt. Substitute salt-free chicken broth for all or some of the water to enhance the taste. Add 1 stick of cinnamon to the liquid at the beginning of the cooking process. A few strands of saffron may also be added at the beginning.

Heartplan Eggplant Spread

1 medium eggplant
1 medium onion, thinly minced
fresh-ground pepper

Pierce skin of eggplant all over with a fork. Bake in a 375°F oven until tender. When cool enough to handle, peel eggplant and remove seeds. Mash flesh well and combine with minced onion. Season with pepper. Chill thoroughly. Remove from refrigerator 15 minutes before serving. Enjoy as a spread for crackers or bread.

Heartplan Baked Fish

Thick-cut firm fish fillets (lemon sole)
Low-fat mayonnaise (Dijon-style mustard and/or herbs can be added for extra flavor)
Bread crumbs or crushed cornflakes

Lightly coat each fillet (both sides) first with mayonnaise and then with crumbs. Place in lightly oiled baking dish. Sprinkle tops of fish with sweet paprika. Bake in 350°F oven about 25 to 30 minutes or until fish easily flakes and crumb coating is golden brown.

Heartplan Chicken Marsala

(serves four)

2 chicken breasts; boned, skinned, halved, and pounded to $1/4$-inch thickness
Fresh-ground black pepper
Flour for dusting
2 tablespoons oil
$1/2$ cup dry Marsala wine
$1/2$ cup saltfree chicken broth
A few drops of fresh lemon juice

Sprinkle both sides of chicken scallops with pepper and coat lightly in flour, shaking off all excess.

Heat 2 tablespoons oil over high heat in a heavy 10- to 12-inch skillet. When the oil is quite hot, not burning, add the chicken pieces. (Do not crowd; if they don't fit, cook in two batches.) Cook scallops 2 to 3 minutes per side, until golden. Don't let them burn or overcook.

Remove scallops from skillet and keep them warm. Remove skillet from heat and quickly deglaze the pan by pouring off all but a thin coating of oil. Return the skillet to the stove. Add the Marsala and bring to a boil over high heat, scraping up any browned particles clinging to the pan. Add the chicken broth and return to a boil; boil for 2 minutes. (The sauce should take on a slightly syrupy consistency.)

Return the chicken scallops to the skillet. Reduce heat to low and baste the scallops with the sauce. Cover skillet tightly with a lid. Simmer for 3 to 5 minutes.

To serve, arrange the scallops slightly overlapping on a platter. Sprinkle with a few drops of lemon and cover with the sauce. You might as well be in Italy!

Heartplan Marinara Sauce

This recipe makes enough sauce for 1 to 1½ pounds of pasta. The sauce is not only delicious and healthful, it also **freezes well** and can be made in large batches for a number of meals.

1 to 2 tablespoons oil
1 large onion, finely chopped
1 clove garlic, finely minced
2 stalks celery, finely chopped
1 carrot, finely chopped
2 teaspoons dried basil
fresh-ground black pepper (to taste)

1 tablespoon dried oregano
¼ teaspoon dried thyme
1 bay leaf
2 pounds Italian plum tomatoes, peeled and seeded (canned tomatoes may be used, but check the label for salt and other additives)
1 tablespoon tomato paste

In a heavy saucepan or 20-inch skillet, heat oil over low flame. Add onion and garlic and sauté for 10 minutes until they are soft, but not brown. Add the carrot and celery and cook for 10 minutes. Stir frequently so the mixture does not burn. Add the basil, oregano, thyme, and bay leaf. Cook, stirring often, for another 5 minutes. Add the tomatoes with their liquid. Raise the heat and bring to a boil. (Optional: break up the tomatoes with the back of a spoon while cooking.) Stir in the tomato paste and black pepper. Cook the sauce over moderate heat for 1 hour. If you like a smooth sauce, pour the sauce into a sieve placed over a large bowl. Press the sauce through the sieve into the bowl and discard any large vegetable particles that remain. Do not puree in a blender or food processor—the sauce will become too liquid.

Other Sources of Healthful Recipes

You can go through any cookbook and modify the recipes so that they are low-fat and low-calorie. Simply keep in mind the basic principles we've set forth in this step. Some publications deserve special mention because they are gold mines of recipes and information about low-fat cooking:

Haas, Dr. Robert,: *Eat To Win*, Signet, New York, 1983.

Eishelman, Ruthe, and Mary Winston, eds.: *The American Heart Association Cookbook*, McKay, New York, 1979. The paperback version is published by Ballantine, New York, 1979.

Claiborne, Craig, and Pierre Franey: *Craig Claiborne's Gourmet Diet*, Times Books, New York, 1980.

Food & Wine magazine. Although dedicated to *haute cuisine*, this publication devotes a special section each issue to adapting a standard recipe to transform it into a low-cholesterol, low-calorie, and low-sodium preparation, all from soup to nuts.

About This Heartplan Program

Let's look at Dr. Rubinstein's cardiac profile after he spent two months on the Heartplan program for great eating:

Age: 43
Height: 5'10"
Weight: 173 lbs.
Blood pressure (average, at rest): 118/78

Average resting pulse: 66/min.
Cholesterol: 160
Triglycerides: 60
HDL as compared to total cholesterol: 28.4% (lowest cardiac risk)

Dr. Rubinstein lost 15 pounds. His blood pressure dropped from being "borderline" high to normal, and his ratio of HDL to cholesterol improved to the point that he had the lowest possible cardiac risk!

Throughout this step, we've refrained from making elaborate lists of foods to eat or not eat. We have avoided the minutiae of counting calories or endless lists of foodstuffs with their milligrams of sodium, protein, carbohydrates, or fat. We've provided you with a few healthful, delicious recipes for eating well and eating right. We've also recommended some excellent books and publications for more information about recipes and food preparation.

Throughout this step, we've avoided the term *diet*, because dieting usually conjures up something temporary, a plan that you abandon once you reach your goals. Instead, we've set forth sensible, easy-to-follow guidelines and principles (and have illustrated them in our 28-day program) to help you rethink food and its relationship to your heart.

We hope this way of viewing food becomes part of your life—for the rest of your life. Here's to a hearty appetite!

Step 6: All about Exercise

Much of what used to be called "aging" isn't aging at all—it's simply disuse! Doctors once thought that the heart's ability to pump blood declined with age and that age also caused body muscle to turn to fat. However, evidence is accumulating that people who exercise into old age maintain youthful cardiovascular and muscle capacities and that those who don't exercise age "normally." The evidence that exercising may prevent or reduce the severity of cardiovascular disease is impressive. In its booklet *Exercise and Your Heart* the American Heart Association says:

> Most of the scientific research has found that, compared to physically active people, inactive people have one-and-a-half to two times the risk of having a heart attack....
>
> The chances of dying immediately after a heart attack are three times greater in physically inactive people.

Exercise may indeed make the consequences of a heart attack much less drastic. Many physicians believe that exercise stimulates the growth of new collateral coronary arteries that can partially compensate for narrowed or blocked vessels. Exercise may enlarge the existing coronary arteries, allowing more blood to pass through them despite some narrowing. Scientific evidence supports these theories.

In addition, experiments at Baylor University have shown that exercise elevates levels of high-density lipoproteins (HDLs) in the bloodstream—these lipoproteins remove cholesterol from the walls of arteries. Elevated HDL levels help to prevent the buildup of atherosclerotic plaque, reducing the risk of developing coronary artery disease.

Physiologists have shown that certain exercises make your heart pump more efficiently, allowing your heart to do its work with less effort. Exercise improves cardiovascular fitness.

Aerobic Exercise

Activities that improve cardiovascular fitness are *aerobic exercises*. Aerobic (literally, with oxygen) exercises increase oxygen supply to your muscles for sustained periods (20 minutes to an hour). They involve rhythmic, repeated movements of large muscle groups. Such exercises are best done steadily, at an effort level below your maximum capacity. Examples include brisk walking, jogging, swimming, bicycling, rowing, and aerobic dancing.

Other exercises, sometimes called *anaerobic*, involve short bursts of energy that don't work the lungs and cardiovascular system as well as aerobic exercise does. Isometric exercise is good for building muscle strength and toning body contours, as anyone knows who works out with weights, but it doesn't promote cardiovascular fitness.

Aerobic exercises should be done at least three times a week for 20 to 30 minutes each session. Start with a warm-up and stretching for 5 to 10 minutes. This is essential to avoid injuries (trying to get a "quick fix" of exercise often results in muscle strains). After warm-up is an aerobic exercise period and, finally, a cool-down period of about 5 to 10 minutes. No matter which exercise regimen you choose, you must approach it gradually. Begin with a few minutes on alternate days, and slowly build up to 30 minutes over a period of weeks or months. For older people, establishing a vigorous program may take as long as six months.

The essential part of each session is the time you spend actually exercising aerobically: jogging, swimming, walking, and so on. Your aim is to engage in this activity so that your heart beats at about 70 to 85 percent of its maximum rate; this 70- to 85-percent rate is called your *target zone*. The average person's maximal heart rate is about 220 beats per minute minus his or her age. Your target zone is 70 to 85 percent of this number. For instance, if you're 50 years old, your maximal heart rate is 170 (220 minus 50). Multiplying this figure by 0.7 and by 0.85 yields a target zone of 119 to 144 beats per minute. Table 1 shows the target zones for various ages, and the figures apply to men and women.

You've probably seen people in sweat suits who take their pulses after jogging. They are most likely checking if their heart rates are within the recommended target zones.

Table 1 Target Zones for Aerobic Exercise

Age	Target Zone	Age	Target Zone
25	136–165	56	114–139
30	133–161	58	113–137
32	131–159	60	112–136
34	129–157	62	110–134
36	127–155	64	109–132
38	126–154	66	107–130
40	126–153	68	106–129
42	125–151	70	105–127
44	123–149	72	103–125
46	122–148	74	102–124
48	120–146	76	100–122
50	119–144	78	99–120
52	117–142	80	98–119
54	116–141		

Note: Many patients, especially those with high blood pressure, take medication that slows the heart rate. The above numbers are not valid for them. An equally good guide is that you should be slightly short of breath so that carrying on a conversation is a little difficult for a few minutes after exercising. You should not be gasping for air!

Most physicians recommend an exercise program for patients who have recovered from a heart attack. For example, exercise groups are an important part of the cardiovascular rehabilitation program for recovering heart attack patients at Danbury Hospital in Danbury, Connecticut. Many patients consider these groups a boon not only because of the exercises, but also because of the sense of camaraderie that group participation engenders.

Before beginning any exercise program, you must consider whether you need a complete medical checkup (including an exercise stress test). We strongly recommend a complete checkup if you fall into one of these categories:

- You are over 40 and have a sedentary life-style.
- You have two or more of the risk factors for heart disease (see Chapter 3).
- You have any diagnosed heart disease.

Any exercise program includes certain dos and don'ts:

- *Do* use common sense! You're not trying to find out how much abuse your body can take.
- *Do* exercise sensibly and regularly—this involves picking a program that you can enjoy and that you will find convenient.
- *Do* enter an exercise program while under a doctor's supervision if you have heart disease or if you are in a high-risk category.
- *Do* enter an organized program at a medical center, a local YMCA, or a community hospital if you are a heart patient. Organized programs provide continuing positive reinforcement to exercise, thus helping you to keep at it.
- *Don't* plunge right in; work up to an appropriate aerobic level for your age, physical condition, and medical history.
- *Don't* become a fanatic. You don't have to be a marathon runner to attain cardiovascular fitness and develop a sense of well-being. Brisk walking is an excellent aerobic exercise for most elderly, previously sedentary people.
- *Don't* exercise in extreme heat or humidity.

What Happened to Jim Fixx?

On a summer afternoon in 1984, Jim Fixx, world-famous running guru, died of a massive heart attack while jogging in Vermont. Many people (especially runners) worried that this ironic event was a warning that too much exercise can be dangerous. Some frequently voiced questions surfaced after Jim Fixx's death:

- Could it happen to me? How can I be sure it won't happen to me? Should I have tests?
- Should we pay more attention to the risks of exercise rather than just its benefits?
- What caused Jim Fixx's death? Does exercise really help prevent cardiovascular disease?

We believe that the evidence overwhelmingly points to exercise as a way to prevent serious heart disease, not cause it. Exercise and sudden death may be connected, but only if you have severe, preexisting coronary atherosclerosis. Remember, a good part of the exercising population already has multiple coronary risk factors, and many people start exercising long after their blood vessels have significant blockage. Some of these people will have heart attacks because they began exercising too late. This is why an exercise stress test is important if you are considering an aerobic exercise program and are in the high-risk category for heart disease.

A recent study of deaths during vigorous exercise found that the victims always had preexisting heart disease. Notably, several weeks before his fatal heart attack Jim Fixx felt a tightening in his throat, but nobody suspected that it might be a signal of underlying coronary artery disease. An examination after his death revealed that Jim Fixx's coronary arteries were severely clogged by atherosclerotic plaque.

Jim Fixx was at high risk for heart disease for a number of reasons. His father had suffered a heart attack at age 35 and died at 43 of heart failure. Before taking up running at age 35, Jim Fixx had smoked two packs of cigarettes a day, was 50 pounds overweight, and had consumed a high-fat diet most of his life. His heredity and early life-style were against him; before he began running, he had severe coronary atherosclerosis.

His dedication to fitness probably kept Jim Fixx alive and healthy much longer than would otherwise have been the case. In general, in families with a history of severe coronary artery disease, the next generation gets sick five or ten years *younger* than the previous one! Jim Fixx modified his risk factors and bettered his father's lifespan by nine years, living until the age of 52. If he had sought medical care when he first experienced symptoms, he might very well be alive today.

Sudden death from heart disease occurs most commonly *at rest*, not during exercise, but these deaths don't make newspaper headlines. There is no question that sudden overexertion can precipitate a heart attack in someone with coronary artery blockage. In fact, the first snowfall each winter usually produces stories of a few unfortunate people who die while shoveling. Such lethal overexertion can easily be avoided. A carefully planned exercise program has little risk.

Most people who engage in sensible and regular aerobic exercise activities feel better emotionally and physically and find that they can more easily maintain an ideal body weight. In addition, they often slim their bodies down to a more healthful and attractive appearance.

A Roster of Aerobic Activities

There is no one best exercise for everyone. Consider your own preferences and the realistic limitations of time and space when you decide on an exercise program. Ideally, a good aerobic activity is fun to do, affords you a certain flexibility in terms of time and weather conditions, can be shared with others (if you prefer it), is not dangerous to your joints and limbs, and provides good cardiovascular conditioning. Our roster includes the most popular aerobic activities.

WALKING

Walking and swimming are the best exercises for the elderly or for previously sedentary middle-aged people. Walking can be especially enjoyable if you live where you can appreciate the changing scenery or, for city dwellers, an ever-changing panoply of people, stores, and activity. Walking is great for aerobic conditioning, but you must move briskly. Walking requires no special preparation, and foot and leg injuries are rare. It can be done alone or with a partner, and it provides flexibility for time and place.

However, if you are young, walking is not strenuous enough to get your heart rate up to your target zone, and it can aggravate chronic foot or leg problems, especially if you walk on pavement. Walking in a large city can expose you to pollutants, and you must choose your terrain with some care. Uphill can be rough.

JOGGING AND RUNNING

Jogging means covering a mile in 10 to 15 minutes; running involves covering the same mile in fewer than 10 minutes. Running and jogging are probably the most popular aerobic exercises in the United States. They are fun, easy, and provide flexibility as to time and place. If you run or jog, make sure to stretch and warm up before you begin!

Some advantages of running and jogging include: You can vary your route; maximum aerobic benefits are obtained for the amount of time and energy you spend; and you burn about 100 calories per mile. This exercise is an excellent adjunct to dieting if you are concerned about weight control.

Some disadvantages include: Running is hard on your knees, shins, ankles, and feet, especially if done on pavement. You must wear good running sneakers, usually expensive, to protect you from injuries. Many orthopedic injuries are caused or worsened by running. Also, some people tend to overdo running since the advent of "marathon consciousness," minimarathons, and other contests that promote competition, resulting in a variety of injuries. Like all outdoor activities, running depends on good weather and the proper terrain.

SWIMMING

Swimming works more large-muscle groups than any other aerobic exercise. You need a large pool, which usually means joining a YMCA or other community center. Swimming is especially good for older people or for those with bone and joint problems, since it places no weight on the lower limbs.

If you swim indoors, you can swim despite bad weather, and thus swimming usually requires joining and traveling to a gymnasium or center. Many people find swimming repeated laps across a pool quite boring. Physical problems such as ear infections, eye irritations, and dry skin from frequent exposure to chlorine may occur.

BICYCLING

Bicycling can be fun-filled exercise; it is an especially good activity with a partner. Bicycling allows a change of scenery as often as you wish, and trauma to the legs and feet is minimal.

As a disadvantage to bicycling, traffic and weather conditions can cause problems and injuries. Also, falls resulting in severe trauma may occur. Your bicycle will require care and maintenance. Some people try to skirt the disadvantages of bicycling by purchasing a stationary bicycle for indoor use, but the program is often abandoned due to boredom. We recommend that you watch television or listen to music when using an exercycle.

AEROBIC DANCING

Aerobic dancing is great for anyone who wants to maintain cardiovascular fitness and who needs a social setting to get started. Once you get into the rhythm of the music, you may feel you can go on forever. Since this can be dangerous, make certain that you begin with a group that is at your own effort level, or you may do too much too soon, causing injuries to your feet, ankles, or lower legs. Once you've built up your endurance, you can do aerobic dance at home on your own.

Final Considerations

Other forms of aerobic exercising include cross-country skiing, using a minitrampoline, rowing, race-walking, vigorous hiking, rope-jumping, running in place, sustained "jumping jacks," and even some weight programs (Nautilus and others). Cross-country ski machines are excellent for cardiovascular conditioning, but they are expensive and require space.

Sports such as softball, bowling, and golf are fun, but they are not aerobic. They may provide many other benefits, but they do not provide cardiovascular conditioning.

Whichever program you choose, begin moderately, and preferably under supervision. This is especially important if you are out of shape, lead a sedentary life, are over 40, or are a high-risk candidate for heart disease. If you have had a heart attack, you should begin under the supervision of your physician.

You may wish to read more about aerobics. We recommend *The New Aerobics* by Kenneth H. Cooper (Bantam, New York, 1970).

Whichever aerobic exercise you choose, whether you do it alone or with other people, whether you exercise in combination with team sports or not, the investment of time and energy will pay great dividends. You will most likely look and feel better than you have in years. And your heart will know the difference.

Step 7: Relaxation

Traditionally, relaxation is any activity that promotes a sense of inner tranquility and well-being, which can be anything from reading a book to watching a favorite television program. As you can no doubt infer, we regularly advise our patients to find outlets for their creative, intellectual, and emotional needs. We also advise patients to set aside time for loafing. Some people have problems doing "nothing"; if left unoccupied by some activity, their minds wander, reviewing the day's troubles and hassles. For these people, doing nothing can be counterproductive, because it leads to more worrying about various problems.

When you're under stress, your muscles become tense, your breathing quickens, your heart beats more rapidly and forcefully, and your blood pressure rises. Your body secretes more adrenaline, your cholesterol level rises, and a variety of other bodily changes occur. In other words, the entire repertoire of fight-or-flight mechanisms is flung into motion.

Relaxation refers to specific ways to "deprime" your fight-or-flight response, especially your cardiovascular system's involvement. Relaxation sets into gear the opposite of these stressful bodily responses, lowering your blood pressure, slowing your heart rate, and promoting a general sense of well-being and restfulness.

How to Undo the Fight-or-Flight Response

Two scientifically proven procedures for depriming the bodily responses elicited by the fight-or-flight posture are progressive

Step 7: Relaxation

relaxation and relaxation response. These two methods of relaxation are both the most popular and the most misunderstood.

Progressive relaxation involves the body's voluntary muscles (those over which you have conscious control, such as your leg and arm muscles). It is practiced lying down in a quiet room. The subject is taught to relax as fully as possible, assuming a totally passive state. Mental images of any kind can induce slight (yet measurable) levels of muscle tension, especially of the face muscles. Subjects are taught to recognize minute contractions of any muscles and avoid them through even deeper relaxation. This method requires a certain amount of instruction by a psychiatrist or other medical therapist, and can be expensive.

The *relaxation response* has achieved wide popularity because of the writing of Dr. Herbert Benson. He coined the term, and his excellent book *The Relaxation Response* (Avon, 1976) should be read by anyone who wishes to learn this easily mastered technique. Our explanation, borrowed from Dr. Benson, will briefly describe how relaxation response works. For a deeper discussion of its background and of the scientific evidence supporting this method, we highly recommend Dr. Benson's informative and readable book.

The physiologic changes of the relaxation response are associated with an altered state of consciousness—here *consciousness* simply refers to a level of awareness ranging from deep unconsciousness to hyperalertness. An "altered state" refers simply to a kind of awareness that is not frequently experienced. Although it isn't strange or abnormal, this consciousness doesn't happen by itself; you must purposely evoke it within your mind through meditation.

For many people, the term *meditation* conjures up images of Tibetan priests, Christian monks, and exotic cults—reclusive people contemplating their god and other spiritual matters. However, there is nothing mystical, philosophical, or religious about the meditation used in the relaxation response technique, although many religions have used meditation throughout the ages.

The relaxation response counteracts everyday stresses through *focusing your mind*. The basic components necessary to bring forth the relaxation response are:

Step 7: Relaxation 147

1. *A Quiet Environment* with as few distractions as possible
2. *A Mental Device* to shift the mind from external distractions. This can be a sound, a word, or a phrase you repeat silently (in meditation, this is called a "mantra"). The repeated sound or word helps keep your mind from wandering. Attention to your normal rhythmic breathing enhances your focusing on the repetition of this sound or word.
3. *A Passive Attitude.* You must keep returning to the repetition of this one word or phrase, even if distracting thoughts enter your mind. These other thoughts don't mean you are performing the technique incorrectly.
4. *A Comfortable Position.* This is important so that there is no muscular tension. Simply stay relaxed; most people find the sitting position best, though the relaxation response can be brought forth in the lying position too.

Here is how it works:

Sitting with your eyes closed, begin relaxing your muscles, starting at your feet and progressing up to your face.

Breathing through your nose, say a word (for instance, "One") silently to yourself. Ignore any distracting thoughts that may come to you; simply breathe in and out, repeating "One" silently to yourself (between breaths) and keep relaxing all your muscles. If you have a distracting thought, refocus your concentration on the word "One" and keep repeating it to yourself between the rhythm of your breathing. It's as simple as that. Don't "work" at it and don't worry if thoughts pop into your mind ... just refocus on "One" ... "One" ... "One" ...

This relaxation mode should be continued for 10 to 20 minutes, twice each day. For some reason, a recent meal interferes with the ability to achieve the relaxation response, so don't do it until two hours after your last meal. Some people prefer a quiet environment to regularly use for relaxation; others can evoke the relaxation response almost anywhere, on a train or subway or even while waiting for a traffic light to change. Of course, under this circumstance, they can do it for only a minute or so at a time.

Scientific evidence clearly points to the relaxation response as a potent way to deprime the body's fight-or-flight mechanism.

Dr. Benson's studies are very convincing. People who practice this relaxation technique achieve a lowering of blood pressure, a slowing of their pulses, and they consume less oxygen during their 10- to 20-minute relaxation period.

People who regularly practice the relaxation response experience a real drop in their blood pressure readings throughout the entire day, not only during the relaxation period. Those who stop practicing the relaxation response soon discover that their blood pressure returns to previous higher levels. This is certainly a powerful testament to the heart-mind connection.

The relaxation response can be used whenever you encounter a stressful situation. People who benefit most from this application are those who target a specific stressful situation. By practicing the relaxation response when they face the problem, they deprime their stress reactions.

Another useful application is to fantasize about a stress you expect you will encounter. Then practice the relaxation response for 10 to 20 minutes to deprime your fight-or-flight response. Over time, you can desensitize yourself to this specific stress even before you encounter it.

Not only does the technique defuse the fight-or-flight mechanisms that stress sets into motion, but also most people who regularly use this relaxation technique report feelings of calm and well-being throughout their daily lives.

No particular ability or aptitude is needed to practice the relaxation response successfully. Nor is any special course of instruction necessary. The basic principles are simply those described. Every human being is capable of experiencing the relaxation response.

We prefer the relaxation response over other ways of achieving relaxation, such as hypnosis or biofeedback, for several reasons. It's cheaper because you don't need an instructor or a course. It doesn't involve any equipment, as biofeedback does, and you can learn it on your own. And it hasn't been associated with magic or with the bizarre, as has hypnosis.

The evidence supporting the beneficial effects of the relaxation response is very convincing. Studies have shown that regular use of this technique results in a sense of inner calm and lower blood pressure. Try it!

Step 8: To Stop Smoking

William Bolin, a 51-year-old man, came for a consultation because of chest pain that occurred whenever he exerted himself. The pain, a dull ache beneath his breastbone, had been present for three weeks and was getting worse. A complete examination indicated that his heart was not getting enough oxygen during periods of exertion. Mr. Bolin had angina pectoris.

Coronary angiography revealed that his disease was severe, but Mr. Bolin was afraid to have coronary artery bypass surgery. He chose medical therapy with risk-factor modification.

He began losing weight and used medication, which brought quick relief, whenever he had chest pain. He lost 10 pounds in three weeks, but his chest pains now occurred with even less exertion than before. In fact, at a wedding a week earlier, chest pain had forced him to sit down after only a few seconds of slow dancing with his wife.

During an office visit with both Bolins, Mrs. Bolin expressed some concern. She couldn't understand why her husband's treatment plan wasn't working. He'd modified his diet, he had stopped smoking (he'd smoked two packs of cigarettes a day for 30 years), and he was trying to reduce the stresses in his life. The couple left the office worrying that Mr. Bolin might have to undergo coronary artery bypass surgery if things didn't change.

At his next visit one month later, Mr. Bolin was very dejected. He and his wife had gone to a dinner dance for the New Year holiday, and he had again tried to dance. To his profound disappointment, he was forced to stop after a short time. The mildest exertion brought on chest pains. Besides worrying that he might have a full-scale heart attack, Mr. Bolin now felt that he was "becoming a cripple."

A thorough review of his treatment program was not very revealing. Mr. Bolin had lost even more weight and was taking his medication properly. Yet his symptoms were worse. The thought of open-heart surgery frightened and depressed him, and Mr. Bolin now saw his options narrowing. What could he do?

Mr. Bolin did not keep his next appointment. A telephone conversation with his wife revealed that Mr. Bolin was on the verge of giving up; he was depressed and could see no reason to visit the doctor, since "it was the same old story." His chest pains had continued as before, forcing him to give up even the mildest activities. Mrs. Bolin was worried about her husband's physical and emotional state, and she promised to try to convince her husband to visit the doctor again.

At his next visit, things were better. Mr. Bolin was able to climb a flight of stairs (slowly) with minimal chest pain and he was in better spirits. His treatment seemed to be paying off.

One week later he returned to the office and was feeling great. He and his wife had attended a charity fund-raiser where there had been square dancing. The couple had danced for 20 minutes at a stretch and Mr. Bolin had no chest pain. They had danced three times during the fund-raiser, and Mr. Bolin felt great. It seemed a miracle.

Somewhat sheepishly, Mr. Bolin revealed the secret of his sudden improvement. He had *not* given up cigarettes at first! He'd been smoking heavily at work and sneaking cigarettes at home. The prospect of open-heart surgery made Mr. Bolin realize that cigarettes could kill him, and he gave them up.

Within 24 hours, he began to feel better; by the third day without cigarettes, he could climb stairs without resting. After 10 cigarette-free days, the Bolins attended the fund-raiser where they square-danced. By then, Mr. Bolin had no chest pains, even with vigorous exertion. His symptoms were gone!

Mr. Bolin's case illustrates certain important points: The first is that the risk factors for heart disease form a complicated mosaic. No doubt, heredity, diet, his weight, blood pressure, stress, and smoking all made contributions to his angina pectoris. But for Mr. Bolin, smoking was the critical factor; it was the one thing that tipped the scales and brought on his angina.

Mr. Bolin's case illustrates what most people who smoke know all too well; smoking cigarettes is a physical and psychological addiction that is very difficult to break. Even when faced with potentially dire consequences, some people find it hard to break the habit. We know some patients stricken with heart disease who continued smoking even while recovering in the hospital!

Mr. Bolin didn't want to acknowledge that cigarette smoking was truly dangerous. He modified other risk factors (diet, stress reduction), but somehow he thought that "one more" cigarette—another week, another month, another year of smoking—would not harm him. Psychiatrists call this *denial*: When people don't want to acknowledge something, they pretend it isn't there or that it doesn't matter.

All smokers use denial. After all, everyone knows that smoking is a major contributor to heart disease, lung cancer, and a variety of other serious ailments. Yet millions of people (many in the high-risk groups for heart disease) continue to smoke. They don't think about the consequences, or, if they do, they tell themselves, "It won't happen to me," or "Someday I'll stop, but not right now."

Mr. Bolin's case also illustrates the self-destructive behavior of people who smoke heavily. Such people often find it very difficult to commit themselves to a decision favoring life over the possibility of disease and death!

Cigarette Addiction

We're not going to give you a step-by-step routine to help you stop smoking. There are many programs for that, and we'll direct you to a few. We will give you some general thoughts and guidelines to help you overcome this addiction.

Addiction is a physical and emotional dependence on a substance such that you must maintain a certain level of intake to feel normal. Giving up an addictive substance brings on withdrawal symptoms (physical and emotional). Addiction induces a craving that has a compulsive, overpowering quality; the addict must use the substance in a certain (sometimes ever-increasing) amount to feel satisfied. Addiction is a state of ongoing intoxication in which your behavior is partly ruled by need for the substance.

Anyone who has ever tried to give up cigarettes recognizes the definition of addiction. It also applies to other drugs such as heroin, cocaine, and alcohol.

Thinking of yourself as an addict who has lost control over part of your life is unpleasant. Even more sobering is the undeniable truth that cigarette smoking is perhaps the most detrimental abuse you can ever inflict on your body. It is a slow form of suicide.

If you have developed angina pectoris or have had a heart attack, *you must stop smoking*. Continuing is tantamount to suicide. If you wish to avoid heart disease, don't smoke. Nine out of ten men with severe coronary disease at a young age are smokers! For young people, cigarette smoking is the major—and most modifiable—coronary risk factor.

In our experience, giving up cigarettes is easier for people who have developed heart disease than for those who are still symptom-free. Relinquishing a well-entrenched addiction is less difficult if you have had a brush with death.

People who give up cigarettes often replace the oral gratification of smoking with eating more, and they often gain weight. Some fear that this weight gain is as harmful as the smoking habit. In truth, most people who quit smoking do gain some weight—about 10 pounds—which levels off in a few months. The dangers of this minimal (and temporary) weight gain don't begin to approach the benefits of not smoking.

Another difficulty with quitting smoking is that smokers must deprive themselves of a tangible pleasure in return for an intangible reward. This is especially hard if they aren't certain that dire consequences—namely, heart disease—will occur.

People who successfully stop smoking exhibit a very important characteristic—they make a resolute and total commitment to life. Yes, they know they will feel temporarily deprived and will suffer addiction withdrawal. They also know that once they do stop, they will *never* smoke another cigarette. They reach a point in their lives where they decide to undo self-destructiveness, confident that they will never return to their addiction.

Thus the solace we offer to someone who wants to quit but who finds the going rough is one word: Life. Others—people who quit only to resume smoking—never cross that threshold of commitment to life. They never abandon the privilege of self-destruction. They make a tentative effort to break their addiction, consoling themselves that they can always return to cigarettes if the going gets rough. Even as they declare that they've smoked their last cigarette, they cannot truly imagine a cigarette-free life. Those who conjure up a comforting image of themselves smoking six months later always go back.

Any method you use to stop smoking will fail unless you make this fundamental commitment to your own life and well-being. All the tips, hints, and programs in the world will be exercises in futility unless you make this deep personal transition toward a health-oriented future—toward life. People who give up cigarette smoking often profoundly change their view of their lives, sometimes completely unconsciously.

One thing is certain. People who quit smoking live longer and healthier lives than those who continue to smoke—even if those who quit had smoked for years. By quitting, they gradually rid their bodies of the noxious effects of nicotine and other chemicals produced by cigarette smoke.

Although statistics convincingly show that cigarette smoking causes people to die early, no one has yet isolated the ingredient in cigarette smoke that actually causes damage to the heart. Perhaps ex-smokers live longer than smokers because they are doing more than simply avoiding deadly toxins produced by cigarette smoke. They may also be making fundamental personality changes.

We often speculate that smokers have personality traits that are injurious (even deadly) to their health. We've seen many cigarette smokers with potent, self-destructive and self-punishing personal traits coupled with certain type A behaviors. Is cigarette smoking only a symptom of these underlying traits? Perhaps giving up cigarettes merely reflects deeper emotional changes that result in less wear and tear on their hearts! Time and research will hopefully tell.

How to Stop Killing Yourself

Once you've made up your mind to quit, you must prepare for the withdrawal symptoms evoked by the addictive components of cigarette smoke. There is no quicker or more dramatic way to kick the habit than by quitting "cold turkey," but this requires a certain resolve. Rest assured that the withdrawal symptoms (some mild restlessness, a periodic craving for a cigarette, irritability, and, for some people, transient lightheadedness) will quickly pass. After ten days, the nicotine in your system has dissipated, and withdrawal then involves the psychological and social components of your addiction.

A cup of coffee, a glass of wine, and various social and psychological settings may trigger a craving for a cigarette. If you've dedicated yourself to a program for life, these minor, habit-induced cravings will not be overpowering. You may be surprised after two weeks how the yearning will disappear. (People who report continual cravings for months or years haven't committed themselves to a cigarette-free life. They are waiting for the first opportunity to reach for a cigarette.) We speak from our knowledge of many patients' reactions to stopping smoking *and* from personal experience, since one of us (Dr. Rubinstein) is an ex-smoker who was addicted for 17 years.

Many people don't feel confident that they can kick the habit alone; they prefer to make a genuine attempt in the company of other people so they can feel less isolated in this crucial health and life-changing effort. The following are some organized stop-smoking programs:

THE AMERICAN CANCER SOCIETY

The American Cancer Society has offices throughout the United States. You can locate the nearest stop-smoking program by calling your local chapter. All group settings offer a behavior-modification program along with peer support for quitting. Groups of 20 to 25 people are led by trained ex-smokers. Quitting is gradual, and the groups meet twice a week for up to ten sessions. An ex-smokers club meets twice a month for those who have completed the program. The American Cancer Society has the most widespread and comprehensive stop-smoking programs available. The organization claims a success rate of 30 percent. (The *success rate* in most stop-smoking programs is the percentage of participants who are still not smoking at the end of one year.) The fee varies from $5 to $35.

You may also contact the national headquarters of the American Cancer Society for more information about stop-smoking programs or for literature about quitting. Their address is 90 Park Avenue, New York, N.Y., 10016; their telephone number is (212) 559-8200.

THE AMERICAN HEART ASSOCIATION

Local chapters of the American Heart Association offer stop-smoking programs in various locations throughout the United States. Contact your local office to locate the one nearest you.

THE AMERICAN LUNG ASSOCIATION

Not as widespread as the American Cancer Society, this organization offers stop-smoking programs in selected locations throughout the United States. Look through your telephone directory for the chapter nearest you.

SMOKENDERS

One of the oldest stop-smoking programs available, Smokenders claims a success rate of over 80 percent. Graduates of the program moderate the six-week course. Behavior modification and support techniques are used. Smoking stops at a cutoff date, and the sessions then help participants to adjust to a nonsmoking life-style. Smokenders programs are widely available throughout the United States. The national telephone number is (800) 528-3462. The fee is $295. You get a discount if you introduce a friend to the program.

SEVENTH-DAY ADVENTISTS

Seventh-Day Adventists offer stop-smoking programs in certain cities where Seventh-Day Adventist churches are located. The approach is cold turkey, and participants meet in five daily 90-minute sessions. The program is nondenominational and claims a 30 percent success rate. Locate a Seventh-Day Adventist church in your telephone directory and then inquire if a stop-smoking program is available in your community. There is usually no fee.

OTHER PROGRAMS

Stop-smoking hypnosis programs are offered by various therapists throughout the country. Hypnosis must be done with a trained and skilled practitioner in group sessions or individually, although this can become expensive. Your telephone directory will list whatever hypnosis services and counseling centers are available in your area. Fees vary depending on the course of treatment you choose.

Nicotine chewing gum is now available to help you stop smoking. Nicorette, available by prescription, contains 2 milligrams of nicotine per piece and can be chewed whenever a quitter feels the craving for a cigarette. This can help diminish withdrawal symptoms of nicotine deprivation. When used in conjunction with a stop-smoking program, the gum proves about 50 percent effective.

If you are mechanically inclined, filtered cigarette holders are available. Use of a progressively more absorbent filter over a few days will diminish the amount of tar and nicotine you inhale so that quitting completely will be easier.

If you have tried to stop smoking and failed many times in the past, take heart. Statistics indicate that the more often you try quitting, the more likely you are to succeed. No matter which program you try, only your motivation and commitment to a better life will make you a nonsmoker.

The following free publications are available by contacting the organization indicated:

About Your Heart and Smoking, American Heart Association Publication 1979 51-037-A; available from the National Center, 7320 Greenville Avenue, Dallas, Texas, 75231.

Calling It Quits, U.S. Department of Health, Education and Welfare Publication (NIH) 79-1824, 1979; available from the National Cancer Institute, Bethesda, Maryland.

Clearing the Air, U.S. Department of Health, Education and Welfare Publication (NIH) 79-1647, 1979; available from the National Cancer Institute, Bethesda, Maryland.

Step 9: Your Medical Program

If you have angina pectoris or hypertension or have had a heart attack, you will need a sound medical program to ensure your future well-being. Recent developments in the treatment of coronary heart disease make your outlook better than ever if you lead a sensible life-style and follow a medical program that is geared to your needs. At the center of any medical plan is your relationship with your physician, because it can influence what you think and feel and how you deal with your disease. In other words, your relationship with your doctor can affect your entire life.

You and Your Physician

The foundation of any good relationship rests on the willingness of the participants to communicate with each other. Good communication is as important in your dealings with your doctor as it is in any situation. Keep this in mind when choosing a physician. You must have confidence in your doctor, and you should like her or him as a person.

Above all, your physician should be willing to talk with you and answer any questions about your condition and its treatment. A physician truly interested in you will welcome the chance to discuss your misgivings or concerns.

Patients sometimes fear that asking questions or voicing concerns imposes on their doctor's time or somehow questions his or her professional competence. Nothing could be further from the truth! You must feel free to ask questions about your disease, its causes, diagnosis, and recommended treatment. Your doctor should help you understand everything you need to know, including the purpose of any prescribed medication. Ignorance of these issues makes compliance with your treatment plan less likely. Abandoning the treatment plan, especially when medication causes side-effects, can have disastrous results.

For instance, patients with hypertension may question the need for medication. After all, hypertension is a symptomless disease, producing no pain or discomfort until the disease has caused irreparable damage to the cardiovascular system and sometimes a heart attack or stroke. Such patients, feeling absolutely fine even as their high blood pressure does its damage, may understandably be reluctant to take the prescribed medication unless a doctor carefully explains how elevated blood pressure hastens atherosclerosis, overworks the heart, and eventually weakens the heart muscle. The doctor must explain the importance of medication that will prevent these disastrous long-term effects, even to a patient who feels fine and sees no present need for medication. Here, communication between doctor and patient is vital!

There are other crucial aspects to your relationship with your physician. Your doctor should take a preventive approach to your condition. Doctors are rarely trained to think in terms of prevention; from the outset of medical school they are taught to treat or cure diseases, not prevent them. If you already have heart disease, prevention means taking steps to keep the condition from worsening. If you do not have heart disease, obviously prevention aims to avoid its development.

To help prevent or minimize heart disease, your physician should encourage you to embrace the various steps of Heartplan:

- Stop smoking.
- Reduce your intake of cholesterol and saturated fats.

- Exercise regularly.
- Discuss any emotional problems at home or at work that cause you undue stress or anxiety and that may be injurious to your health and well-being. Counseling or a stress-management program should be recommended if these problems interfere with your capacity for enjoyment, especially if worrying about your condition prevents you from participating in work or social activities, including a normal sex life.
- Learn to deal with stress appropriately.
- Discuss any concerns you have about your condition and its treatment.
- Communicate with your partner. Discuss any concerns he or she may have about your condition, its treatment, and how it affects your relationship. Your doctor should ask to meet periodically with both you and your partner. If he doesn't ask, suggest it to him.

Your physician should be a working model of good, sound cardiovascular fitness. In other words, your doctor should believe in and live by the recommendations he or she offers in your treatment. If your doctor is 40 pounds overweight and lights a cigarette while discussing your Heartplan, you're getting a not-so-subtle wink of the eye along with the good advice. The mixed message says, "You don't *really* have to bother with these things. Go right on living the same life of excess and you'll be fine." This unspoken advice can kill you. Find a physician who is a good role model, because you'll need your doctor's psychological support to help you make necessary life-style changes.

Similarly, choose a physician who doesn't make you or your partner feel that you are now a semi-invalid. Your doctor should advocate a sensible roster of activities that ensure as full and rich a life as possible. Advising you to accept less than that is the stuff of invalidism. Avoid it! Remember, with modern medical therapy, nearly all heart disease symptoms can be prevented or controlled.

Psychiatrists know that sometimes the most important part of any patient's treatment is the relationship between the patient and the physician. A good relationship can enhance the treatment, and a bad relationship can cause treatment to fail. Thus your relationship with your doctor can be the most critical part of your medical program, working for you or against you. It can influence you to follow sound advice and properly take medication or to ignore the advice and medication and risk your life.

Remember, if you have heart disease, you and your doctor are a team with the common goal of helping you deal with the disease so that you can live as full a life as possible. If you are not a patient, your goal is to avoid becoming one while living a full life.

Your Medical Treatment

The foundation of therapy for coronary heart disease combines a low-fat diet, no smoking, stress reduction, and an exercise program. Such a program prevents the progression of atherosclerosis and is essential for arresting the disease. Progression of the disease beyond a certain point causes symptoms such as angina pectoris and engenders the possibility of a heart attack.

The next line of treatment is medication, which is used mainly to control symptoms. It has little effect on the underlying course of the disease. Thus medication is important if you have symptoms, but your future well-being depends almost entirely on risk-factor reduction. Research clearly shows that the best way to prevent a second heart attack is to stop smoking. Managing stress more effectively is second, and a healthy diet and use of beta-blocker medication run a close third. Angioplasty or surgery is the treatment used last; it is reserved for very severe cases.

Two patients rarely have the same treatment plan. Whether a medication or a combination of medicines is appropriate will depend on your age, your specific heart condition, its severity, your weight, your diet, how well you tolerate medicine, and various other factors.

Here is a roster of medications used frequently in treating heart disease:

NITROGLYCERINE

Nitroglycerine is an effective medication for relieving the chest pain of angina pectoris. Tablets placed under the tongue are rapidly absorbed and usually stop angina pain in minutes. Nitroglycerine lowers blood pressure; dilates the coronary arteries, allowing more blood to get to the heart; and decreases the heart's work load.

Because sublingual (beneath-the-tongue) nitroglycerine's effects last only about half an hour, long-acting nitrates have been developed. Some, such as Sorbitrate and Isordil, last up to two hours when taken by mouth. Other preparations are available in ointment form that is absorbed through the skin.

BETA BLOCKERS

Beta blockers are excellent medications for the patient who has both hypertension and angina pectoris. One medication can be used to treat both diseases. Inderal was the first medication of this kind, but several newer beta blockers, including Tenormin, Lopressor, and Corgard, have become popular because they cause fewer side-effects.

Beta blockers block the effects of the sympathetic nervous system on the heart; they prevent the fight-or-flight message from getting to the heart, avoiding an unnecessarily fast or irregular rhythm. They also reduce the work load of the heart by decreasing the oxygen it needs, thereby making the heart pump more efficiently. Beta blockers reduce the chance of death after a heart attack in patients who have survived a first heart attack.

DIGITALIS

Some form of digitalis has been available since 1785, and it is still a primary weapon in controlling congestive heart failure. Digitalis increases the strength of heart muscle, making it a stronger and more efficient pump. It relieves symptoms of congestive heart failure such as breathlessness (dyspnea), caused by fluid buildup in the lungs, and ankle swelling (edema). The most widely used preparation is Lanoxin, whose generic name is digoxin.

ANTIHYPERTENSIVES

Antihypertensives work by various mechanisms within the cardiovascular system to lower blood pressure in people with hypertension. Some of the better-known preparations are Aldomet, Minipress, and Apresoline. Other kinds of medications (such as beta blockers and diuretics) are also used to lower blood pressure. Many hypertensive patients can avoid drugs by following a program of weight reduction, exercise, and stress management.

DIURETICS

Diuretics remove fluid from the body by increasing urine output. Increased urine output helps rid the body of excess salt and water, and the result is lower blood pressure. Diuretics are also used to treat the symptoms of congestive heart failure such as edema and dyspnea. Diuretics tend to deplete the body of potassium, so patients taking diuretics should eat foods high in potassium (bananas, orange juice, and apricots). Some well-known diuretic preparations are Diuril, Hydrodiuril, Aldactone, Dyazide, Hygroton, and Lasix.

CALCIUM BLOCKERS

Calcium blockers are a new class of medications that have been available only a few years. They lower blood pressure, dilate the coronary arteries, and slow the heart rate. Commonly used calcium blockers are Procardia, Calan, and Cardizem.

MEDICATIONS TO LOWER CHOLESTEROL AND TRIGLYCERIDES

For most patients, strictly limiting the intake of fat lowers blood cholesterol to acceptable levels. Use of medication to lower cholesterol levels should be reserved for patients with very high cholesterol that has not been reduced by a strict low-fat diet. Most of these medications taste terrible and have unpleasant side-effects.

TRANQUILIZERS

Physicians may prescribe various tranquilizers for patients who feel constantly stressed or nervous. We prefer the stress management techniques we have described. We also recommend exercise and the relaxation response, as outlined in Heartplan. Tranquilizers can be both physically and psychologically addictive and are sometimes abused by patients. Some popular tranquilizers are Valium, Librium, Serax, Xanax, and Ativan. If nonstop stress is a continuing problem, seeking emotional counseling is probably a better answer than the frequent use of tranquilizers.

Choosing a Medication

Medications are potent chemicals! All can cause side-effects of some kind or another, although most side-effects are minor. In a small percentage of patients, though, they can be troublesome and very unpleasant. Side-effects are rarely permanent or irreversible, and they can be eliminated with reduced dosages or shifts to other medicines. If you experience side-effects, inform your doctor; reducing or eliminating your dosage on your own is very dangerous. A mere telephone call to your doctor will ensure that side-effects are eliminated!

Choosing the right medication may take a while, and you may have to try several before you find one that doesn't cause side-effects. This process requires close cooperation with your doctor. Although finding the right medicine may take a while, the final result can be well worth the effort, since the medication may make an enormous difference in your future well-being. Remember, you may have to take the medication for many years.

In some instances, you may have to accept occasional side-effects caused by your medication. Living with minor side-effects may mean trading one symptom for another.

Your treatment requires periodic checkups to prevent or minimize the side-effects of some medications. A few drugs have delayed side-effects, and some side-effects can be detected only by a physical examination or a laboratory test. Checkups may include a physical examination, electrocardiogram, and other tests that are indicated.

In addition to monitoring the effects of your medication, your doctor should encourage you to keep up with your Heartplan and should help you assess any ongoing stresses in your life. Most patients need frequent reminders about the importance of diet, exercise, and stress reduction in their lives. These crucial components of Heartplan are easily forgotten once you are feeling well.

Remember that your emotional state is as important as the physical aspects of your situation, since these two elements are intimately connected. In a very real way, optimism, laughter, a sense of inner calm, and a modicum of contentment are the very best medicines.

If You Have a Heart Attack

A heart attack can be terrifying. The sudden onset of symptoms is followed by the urgent atmosphere of an ambulance, the emergency room, and finally, a coronary care unit (CCU). An unreal quality pervades, and the entire experience is one of threat, fear, and isolation.

Your initial contacts in the CCU are with the staff, your physicians, and your family. Because you have little contact with other patients, you may even feel as though you are the only patient in the hospital. An excellent way to begin the transition from the isolation of a CCU back to normal life is through a group setting.

At Danbury Hospital, a rehabilitation nurse visits with you and your family when you are well enough. Topics discussed range from the return to work after discharge to certain life-style changes. Your doctor and the rehabilitation nurse explain how your heart disease developed and what important life-style changes will help you stay healthy. Some of this discussion takes place on an individual basis, but much of the inpatient rehabilitation program uses a group setting.

Group sessions early in the rehabilitation program can help you develop a perspective about your current situation and your plans for the weeks, months, and even years ahead. Patients hear lectures, view videotapes about heart disease, and discuss how to change life-style mistakes such as smoking and overeating. After discharge, rehabilitation is continued with group exercise sessions and educational programs.

Dr. Richard H. Rahe and his associates at the San Diego Health Research Center studied group sessions for post-heart attack patients. Patients participated in six group sessions both before and after discharge from the hospital. The group emphasis was on altering life-style mistakes considered instrumental in the development of heart disease; the patients focused on changing diets, stopping smoking, and managing life stresses.

The evidence of success in these groups was overwhelming. In a number of trials, Dr. Rahe demonstrated that patients who participated in six group meetings had a 90-percent return-to-work rate after their heart attacks. The usual rate is 50 percent! Follow-up studies revealed that these patients had a very low rate for second heart attacks (even five years later), even though some participants had lapsed back into bad habits such as gaining weight and smoking.

The groups also focused on certain emotional aspects of rehabilitation, and patients who took part in the sessions made crucial psychological adjustments in reducing life-style mistakes that lead to stress reactions. Patients modified two important areas of behavior: they decreased both their sense of time urgency (a type A characteristic) and their tendency to overwork (a Sisyphus trait). These modifications were made in six sessions without deep or probing efforts to understand patients' personalities.

The sessions identified stresses that the patients expected to encounter in daily life and then focused on the ways in which they could modify or eliminate these stresses. More than one-third of the group's time (two to three sessions) was spent rehearsing how patients could cope with stress. For instance, if a patient was worried about how to deal with a particular coworker, that patient would role-play the situation with another patient; thus patients would thoroughly rehearse managing one of the ongoing stresses in their lives even before leaving the hospital.

The most helpful aspect of these sessions is that they encourage people to look at their lives and to realize that overwork, hurrying, and worry about work are long-established—but changeable—habits. We have been very gratified by the reactions of our patients who have participated in group sessions.

> Robert Butler, a bricklayer who had a heart attack on the job, talked about the sessions: "I wasn't sure about it [the sessions] and didn't think it would be for me. I remembered movies where people in groups screamed at each other, stuff like that. It was different, though. We rehearsed situations that would come up on the job, stressful ones, and how we'd handle them. But the big thing was that I saw there were other guys with the same problem."
>
> Scott Renzo, a stockbroker, attended six sessions after his discharge from the hospital. He commented that the group mobilized members back to work and activity:
>
> > "The important thing was that I pinpointed the biggest problem in my life—overwork. Some of the guys were worried they'd never get back to work; but me, I was ready to go the

moment I was out of the CCU. That's the crux of my problem. I used to think nothing of putting in an 80-hour week. And it never got me anything worthwhile. The group began changing that for me.

"And I didn't feel so alone. There were six of us going through the same thing. We were like a family. Now, four years later, three of us still attend an exercise group."

Group sessions have an enormous impact on both the immediate and the long-range prospects of people who take part in them. They address immediate needs by providing emotional support during a crisis. As a transition from the CCU, they can be vital. Simply seeing other people in a similar situation can lessen the fear and sense of isolation that often accompany a stay in the CCU.

Group sessions address your long-range prospects by helping you to change certain life-style mistakes. Organizations such as Weight Watchers and Smokenders successfully use groups to help people alter self-damaging behaviors. Group pressure for members to lose weight and stop smoking can be very powerful. In some groups we have conducted, members actually competed to see who could lose the most weight over the course of the next month! Here, too, simply knowing that other people are trying to alter the same life-style mistakes can help you to do so.

Group sessions also encourage members to recognize and modify stress-inducing attitudes such as time-urgency and workaholism. Unfortunately, few hospitals offer group sessions in stress-management techniques to post-heart attack patients. Most hospitals do, however, have group meetings to help their patients alter mistakes such as smoking, overeating, and lack of exercise. We heartily recommend *any* group setting; the very nature of a group can help you make crucial positive changes. At Danbury Hospital, the Heart Club meets once a month to discuss a relevant topic for any person who has had a heart attack. It provides an important setting for group interactions.

More and more hospitals and cardiac rehabilitation centers are adding group sessions to their programs for patients recovering from heart attacks. If your hospital does not have such an arrangement, ask someone at your local chapter of the American Heart Association about the availability of group meetings. In many programs, psychiatrists are part of the treatment team and conduct group meetings. Rehabilitation nurses and other medical staff are also being trained to participate in these meetings.

The benefits such groups can offer are enormous: They can help change the way you feel about your disease, yourself, and the rest of your life.

PART 3
Anything Else You Need to Know

PART 3

Anything Else You Need to Know

8

Your Sex Life

No topic arouses as much concern for patients as the question of sex after a heart attack or a diagnosis of angina. Myth, misinformation, and distortion abound, maybe because discussing sexual activity is often difficult for both patients and doctors. It isn't at all unusual for cardiac patients to receive no advice or counseling about sex from their physician.

Sometimes a patient's anxiety about sex is part of a general concern about resuming a normal life. After all, a heart attack is indeed a life-threatening event, and angina pectoris is a telling reminder of one's mortality. After such momentous threats, any patient might wonder about new limitations—on work, family life, exercising, or sex.

Because sex is such a charged issue for many people, questions of how, when, or if one can resume or continue normal sexual activity take on special meaning. Unfortunately, doctors and patients rarely discuss sex in an open way—the doctor may be embarrassed or reluctant to bring it up, and a patient, sensing this, may assume that the subject—and perhaps the activity—is strictly taboo. Then the patient leaves the hospital or the doctor's office thinking that his or her sex life has come to an abrupt end. This is completely untrue!

Post-heart attack and angina patients who receive no guidance from their doctors often decide—on their own—that sex is bad for them and must be carefully planned and executed so that it places very little strain on the heart. A number of studies indicate that patients who received little information about sex after a heart attack report a decrease in the frequency and spontaneity of intercourse when and if they resume sexual activity. Many post-heart attack patients report that they have disturbing problems of decreased sexual desire and impotence when they come home from the hospital. Many angina pectoris patients have the same difficulty.

Problems of impotence and decreased desire are not caused by ordinary readjustment difficulties. They stem instead from two common myths about sex and the cardiac patient.

The first myth is that a person suffering from a serious illness should not be sexually active. This belief arises from the popular notion that people should be physically inactive and emotionally passive when recovering from an illness—*any* illness. Once heart disease has been diagnosed, many people expect themselves and are expected by others to assume an invalid's role.

The second myth is that a cardiac patient is liable to suddenly die during intercourse. This fear obviously contributes to the dramatic decline in both frequency and pleasure of intercourse. To a patient who is not fully informed, the idea that sex will tax the heart beyond its capacity may seem logical.

In part this myth comes from the popular ideas that stemmed from the Masters and Johnson studies, which showed a great increase in the work load of the heart during intercourse. But these figures were obtained from observations of college students who engaged in sexual activities with unfamiliar sex partners. Such data are not relevant to older people who have longstanding sexual relationships with a steady partner. For them, the work load placed on the heart is no more than that of climbing two flights of stairs or of walking two city blocks.

Heart attacks during intercourse are rare. The few that have been reported are usually associated with a great deal of emotional stress such as may occur during sex in an extramarital affair. In some cases, an increased physical load may have been placed on the heart because the person had intercourse after eating a heavy meal or drinking far too much alcohol.

A recent study of the heart's response to exercise showed that deaths during treadmill stress tests are extremely rare. Heart rates reached during treadmill stress tests are generally much higher than those reached during sexual intercourse.

Many old-fashioned ideas persist about sex and exercise. These old notions often make patients feel that they are invalids who can never have normal lives no matter how well they feel. Science has disproved these old beliefs, doctors recommend exercise programs for cardiac patients, and sexual activity for patients is no longer considered risky. Rather, sex is beneficial for those who wish to resume or continue a normal life. As a matter of fact, an enjoyable sex life is one of the best ways to reduce ongoing stresses in one's life.

As for sexual intercourse for the cardiac patient, there is no preferred time or position for either partner. The only general rule is that you make certain that you have properly taken any prescribed medication. The only times to avoid intercourse are after eating a heavy meal or drinking alcoholic beverages.

Most post-heart attack patients can resume normal sexual activity a few weeks after returning home from the hospital. In the rare instance of a patient having chest pain or becoming breathless during intercourse, a physician should be notified. Appropriate therapy will almost always prevent these symptoms.

Patients concerned about resuming sexual activity may wish to return to intercourse gradually. They may prefer masturbation at first, followed by a week or two of mutual caressing with their partner. Intercourse can follow later. There is no rule about how to proceed, and there is no "right way" to go about resuming your sex life.

If you have any reservations about resuming your sex life after you leave the hospital, discuss them with your doctor and with your partner. Good communication is essential. Silence and vagueness are to be avoided.

Some medications can interfere with potency. Other medications, including certain antihypertensives, some diuretics, and one or two beta blockers, may cause problems in ejaculation or orgasm for some men and women. However, these problems are usually temporary and can be resolved by a dosage decrease. If the dosage change doesn't help, your doctor can prescribe a different medication that will relieve the difficulty.

Don't be a prisoner of embarrassment or silence. Report any new-found sexual difficulty to your doctor; also discuss it with your partner. Needless worrying and wondering will solve nothing. Sometimes just talking about your concerns makes things better; you may simply be worrying about the possible consequences your situation may have on your sex life. Talk with your doctor.

Sometimes, physicians are not comfortable talking about personal matters or don't feel capable of advising you. Today, medical schools have extensive courses in human behavior, and medical students are much more knowledgeable about sexual behavior than students were years ago. Although some physicians are not comfortable discussing patients' sexual difficulties, younger doctors are getting some training in this important area. However, counseling with a psychiatrist is your best bet if you and your partner experience persistent sexual difficulties.

Today, most cardiac patients start on a graduated exercise program under a doctor's supervision or while attending a cardiac rehabilitation program. Regular exercise is good for your heart and can benefit your sex life as well. Through exercise your heart rate declines, and the heart becomes more efficient. Developing cardiovascular fitness reduces the likelihood that sex—or any reasonable and enjoyable activity—will put a strain on your heart.

9
Living with a Heart Patient

Wife, husband, children, and other close relatives: Heart disease strikes families, not just individuals, and often people close to the patient must make certain adjustments. Since most patients we see with heart disease are married men between 40 and 70 years old, much of what follows pertains to wives. You can alter the advice to fit your specific situation.

Heart disease in any form—for that matter, *any* illness—is a family matter that calls for the pooling of emotional resources between partners and among close family members. Heart disease often requires alterations in diet and life-style that affect the entire family. These changes require a certain amount of cooperation, flexibility and a genuine give-and-take among close family members, especially between husband and wife. Everything we have written in this book applies to a patient's family as well as the patient! For example, patients will find it extremely difficult to give up bad habits if everyone around them continues their bad habits.

Managing Stress

Because stress reduction is so crucial for the well-being of any heart patient, you have to assess frankly your relationship with your spouse. Do conflicts need to be ironed out to reduce stress in your lives? Can enough give-and-take tone down any longstanding problems in the relationship? Can you reinforce your spouse's need to reduce unnecessary stresses without being overly protective? These are difficult questions. Sometimes, partners' best efforts do not succeed, and they actually undo the positive results that both spouses are trying to achieve.

Sharing the Heartplan

Becoming a Heartplan partner will benefit you and your spouse. For instance, one goal is to reduce the intake of saturated fats and cholesterol. Partners must actively participate in this crucial lifestyle change, and you can discover new recipes and help to create less fatty and more exciting meals. If your spouse doesn't want to miss favorite dishes, you can help to modify them (by creative substituting of ingredients) or save them for a rare indulgence. Making these adjustments in your eating and cooking, really, in your thinking, can be challenging and fun while you play a crucial role in your spouse's efforts to live a more healthful life.

Consider participating in your spouse's exercise program—you will discover a wide range of new activities and share new experiences. One wife we know began walking with her husband, who had developed angina pectoris. Six months later, the couple—now retired—enjoyed a brisk, 5-mile walk nearly every day. Activities such as walking, jogging, bicycling, and swimming can be enjoyed as a source of sharing, physically and emotionally, and can benefit each of you.

For some couples, the diagnosis of heart disease brings more than just the negative aspects such as concern about health and longevity. It also provides an opportunity for closeness that may not have been previously apparent.

Many things can influence how well you and your spouse meet the challenges of adjusting to heart disease. Personality makeups affect this adjustment. So will your prior relationship. You both will also be influenced by how the illness affects each of you, other family members, and people outside the family such as friends and colleagues.

An important challenge is to avoid becoming overly protective. Certain forms of overprotectiveness are more common than others. One of the most damaging is to avoid sexual intercourse because you think that sex will strain your partner's heart. Avoiding sex can cause a great deal of anxiety, making any patient feel rejected or "worthless." Rejection is thus added to an already sagging level of self-esteem, since some patients feel that they are falling apart once the diagnosis of heart disease is made. If you have any doubts or questions about sexual activity following a heart attack or the onset of angina pectoris, reread Chapter 8. Discuss openly any additional questions or reservations with your spouse and your spouse's physician.

Preventing your spouse from taking part in any physical activity is a form of overprotectiveness. Exercise is good for the heart.

Another mistake is to warn your partner against any genuine display of emotion, whether it be annoyance, occasional anger, surprise, disappointment, or other feelings. Such feelings are part of anyone's life—because your spouse has heart disease doesn't mean that she or he must now be an emotional robot. Constant warnings and cautions about physical or emotional reactions can be demoralizing and may foster feelings of invalidism. Patients who feel that their lives are constantly scrutinized will feel resentful and engage in damaging recriminations.

You may occasionally have to reinforce advice about reducing unnecessary stresses. The best way for you and your spouse to reach an understanding about these issues is to discuss them openly. Silence invites misunderstanding and resentment.

It's My Fault

We occasionally see a wife who feels guilty because her husband has developed heart disease. Feeling that she somehow caused or contributed to his illness, she may develop sympathetic symptoms such as chest pain, palpitations, or breathlessness, even though she's perfectly healthy. This emotional reaction may reflect on the state of the relationship before the husband became ill. The guilt-ridden wife may even feel, "If only I'd been nicer to him," "If we hadn't argued so often," or, "It's my fault he was overweight and got into trouble," along with other self-punishing accusations.

We tell such a wife that heart disease is the final common pathway of a complicated variety of contributing factors such as heredity, age, stress, diet, and smoking. Some are within any patient's control, whereas others are not. Another crucial point is that as a patient's spouse you probably contributed very little to the illness—but you *can* contribute a great deal to overcoming the heart disease!

The following pages present questions we often hear, along with the advice that is generally most appropriate. Again, alter the content to fit your own specific situation.

Frequently Asked Questions

My husband is 50 years old. Heart disease runs in his family; he smokes cigarettes and has high blood pressure. But he won't go to a doctor. He says things will turn out however they will, and there's nothing he can do about it. What can I do?

This kind of fatalism can be dangerous. Your husband's wish to leave everything to fate means he is leaving his disease and its treatment to fate, which could have grave consequences.

Be forceful and persistent in trying to get him to do what is best for him and the family at this point. You may have to engineer his treatment, because his use of denial and his fatalistic sense of complacency could prove dangerous. The trick, however, is to avoid making the issue a struggle because of the damaging stress that it can cause.

Tell your husband what is disturbing to you about his denial of his illness. The best way to deal with his fatalism is with facts that will be a convincing argument in favor of treatment. You may have to be slightly manipulative here, letting your husband know that the best way he can show his love for you is to get the proper treatment for his disease.

You can also begin helping him make practical changes toward a healthier life-style. If you do the cooking, begin to cut down on fatty foods, cholesterol, and salt. Try making this change an exciting new activity. Be enthusiastic! Be innovative! Try cooking low-fat, low-calorie dishes that are a little exotic. Suggest a mutual activity such as bicycling, walking, jogging, or swimming to help him shed pounds and lower his blood pressure. These activities will be good for you, too! In other words, even without his active cooperation, you can help him begin his Heartplan.

Heart disease is a disease of excess: too much food, fats, stress, smoking, and so on. Your role at this point is to help your husband's awareness grow so that he can live a longer healthier life. If none of this works, you may suggest that you both seek counseling.

My husband developed angina pectoris some time ago. Since the diagnosis, he's working harder than ever. He often forgets his medication and skips his appointments with his doctor. He still gets angry and easily blows up at petty annoyances. I'm very worried. What can I do?

People who minimize things or deny their importance throughout their lives will react to the diagnosis of heart disease in the same way. Your husband may be like many people who fear dependency, passivity, and any kind of enforced limitation of activity. Therefore he isn't complying with medical advice or with his medical program.

In our experience, men with such problems often have an exaggerated idea of the seriousness of their illness. That is, they have a notion that angina pectoris or a heart attack means the "beginning of the end" of a productive, independent life. For such men, complying with a medical program may mean acknowledging the overpowering significance of the illness, which is an intolerable thought.

Such fears are unfounded and are often poorly thought out; they may actually go unrecognized by the patient. It may help for you and your husband to meet with his doctor to discuss these concerns. The chances are that if your husband is told that he can lead a full life with angina, he may not fear its implications as much as he now does. He may have less need to deny his illness and may be more willing to comply with medical advice. Remind your husband that many successful men—Henry Kissinger, Alexander Haig, Norman Cousins, Arthur Ashe, and Craig Claiborne—lead active, vigorous lives in spite of heart disease.

My husband is 56 and had a heart attack last year. He seems physically well now, but he's afraid to do anything. He doesn't work, and he's applying for disability benefits. He doesn't respond to me with a playful cuddle, and our sex life has disappeared. We've lost touch with friends, and he's turned away from everyone. He's not the man I married. What should I do?

Your husband sounds as though he's become a cardiac invalid. For certain patients, their illnesses become part of their entire view of themselves; heart disease may become the most important thing in their lives, dominating and controlling everything. Sometimes a man with sexual problems may use his heart condition to avoid any sexual activity. Or a man who worked for years despite having conflicts about success may use his heart disease as a face-saving retreat from competition for promotion and success. It offers an acceptable form of avoidance.

It's difficult to make specific recommendations without having seen your husband, but his withdrawal from work, social, and sexual activities indicates a poor adaptation to his situation. The longer this problem continues, the better the chances are that it may become deeply entrenched. Go for counseling as a couple—your husband will probably find this easier to accept than individual counseling—so he can better deal with his condition.

My husband has high blood pressure. We've learned over the years that he can control it by losing weight and limiting salt intake. After seeing his doctor, he watches his calories and salt, but after a few weeks, he's back to his old eating habits and he gains weight. How can I get him to stay on a diet?

Try to forget the concept of diet. The very word conjures up thoughts of deprivation, of something temporary and to be abandoned once a certain goal (such as 10- or 20-pound weight loss) is reached. Make a permanent change in the ways you prepare and eat foods; this is part of our Heartplan philosophy.

If you do the cooking, you can do a great deal of creative substituting to prepare delicious, low-calorie, and low-fat meals. Salt substitutes are helpful for salt lovers. Certain foods have a natural taste that approximates saltiness. Use herbs, spices, and flavor enhancers instead of salt, sugar, or fat. Eating differently and healthfully is a matter of educating the family palate to appreciate new, subtle, and interesting tastes. Remember, diets are almost always short-term solutions with short-term results.

My husband is healthy, but he's in the high-risk group for developing heart disease. I prepare low-fat foods at home, but he eats fatty food at lunch every day. Every week, when he goes bowling with his friends, he eats fried food. No matter what I say, it doesn't change. We argue about this a lot. What should I do?

It's commendable that you're aware of the risks for heart disease and that you're doing something to modify them. But there's a problem in this arrangement: Be a partner, not a parent, to your husband. He seems to be rebelling against any restraints that the possibility of heart disease may place on his life, and, in the process, against you. Once you begin to symbolize a parental authority who says no, he may rebel even more, much to his own detriment. This mother-son pattern probably has been part of your relationship in more ways than you've been aware. Search your mind for evidence that it has infiltrated other areas of your lives as well, and make every effort to be less motherly and demanding. The less he has to rebel against, the more he may be willing to protect his own health and well-being.

My husband had a heart attack two years ago. He's doing very well, but there's one problem. He refuses to eat in a restaurant or at friends' homes, and we've become socially isolated. How can I handle this?

Some patients can do too much of a good thing by making an obsession of dieting, or some other aspect of their Heartplan. There's no need for such fanaticism when there are many strategies for eating healthful *and* enjoyable foods. The foremost strategy is cholesterol and calorie banking, which allows for the occasional indiscretion. Even without banking, many restaurants prepare food in healthful ways. With good friends, you may have to make an occasional request, but here too, salads, vegetables and other low-fat choices are usually available.

I've had angina for three years, and my husband has reacted very badly. He constantly worries, smothering me with kindness. I'm beginning to feel like a cripple. How can I handle this?

We have seen some partners overreact to the news that a husband or wife has heart disease. In some cases, the spouse may be preoccupied about what will happen to *him* if he loses his wife. Some husbands begin imagining it's inevitable that their wife will die, and they become frightened. This can result in overcompensation, with fretting and worrying and a kind of smothering solicitousness.

Explore with your husband exactly what he's so worried about. You may find that he's reacting to a fantasy rather than the reality. Once you both discuss the real situation, he may calm down. Openness and honesty are essential. If after this you feel the problem still persists, you should both seek counseling.

My husband is 48 years old and had a heart attack seven months ago. He's doing very well, but our 16-year-old daughter is reacting poorly. She's depressed and worried. How can we handle this?

We often find that people react to the diagnosis of heart disease with the expectation that something terrible will happen, even if the prognosis for recovery and a full life is excellent. This is partly because people are often awed by the thought of a problem with the heart, an organ often endowed with magical meanings.

Your daughter probably has misconceptions about heart disease that are not in step with reality. In other words, she may have a *fantasy* about your husband's problem, one that is much more frightening than the actual situation. Have a frank discussion with her, explaining exactly what is wrong (and what isn't), detailing what is being done and how it will help her father. You should even consider having your daughter discuss this with your husband's physician. Reassurance from an expert is often very valuable.

Vague and poorly defined issues make room for frightening thoughts and distortions. Facts and the simple truth are important, because, in reality, with the proper treatment and life-style changes, a patient's prognosis is usually excellent.

My husband has angina pectoris. Whenever we have a disagreement, he gets chest pains. How can we avoid this?

This is a loaded question. When a spouse has developed angina pectoris or another form of heart disease, most couples should reevaluate some aspects of their relationships. While serious problems may not be avoidable in some marriages, unnecessary stress should be kept to a minimum. Your husband must learn how to handle stress so that it exacts less of a toll from his heart and well-being. Taking a nitroglycerine tablet when stress is anticipated will usually prevent chest pains.

Smoldering conflicts should be explored together and targeted so that he may deal with them in a more adaptive, less harmful way. Your husband's angina pectoris pains inject a new and complicated dimension into your relationship. You must both learn to deal with this. Remember too that he may exploit his condition to make you feel guilty, whenever you disagree.

10
All about Heart Surgery

Early in this century, surgeons would not even think about operating on the heart. Over the years, a few bold experimenters tried certain limited procedures—some successful—but the attempts were few and the results not good.

Today, heart surgery is the most spectacular and controversial aspect of modern medicine. We all read about famous people undergoing coronary artery bypass operations, and lately, the news media have been filled with stories about heart transplants and artificial hearts. In this chapter, we will discuss cardiac surgical procedures and will give you a perspective on these exciting new developments.

The Coronary Bypass

In 1969, Dr. Rene Favaloro developed an operation that has changed the face of modern cardiac surgery. Using a saphenous vein from the leg, he bypassed (went around) a clogged portion of coronary artery, so that blood could go from the aorta to the heart tissue, circumventing the blocked portion of the artery. A good analogy is the rerouting of automobile traffic to a freeway that circles the clogged streets of a congested, inner city (see Figure 5).

The increase in incidence of this operation has been fantastic: 13,000 were done in 1970; more than 200,000 coronary artery bypass grafts (CABGs) were done in 1984. The operation is now the medical leader in terms of equipment and personnel, hospital space, training programs, and total surgical revenues throughout the United States. It has been popularized in the media, aggrandized by the medical profession, and is the epitome of sophisticated medical technology.

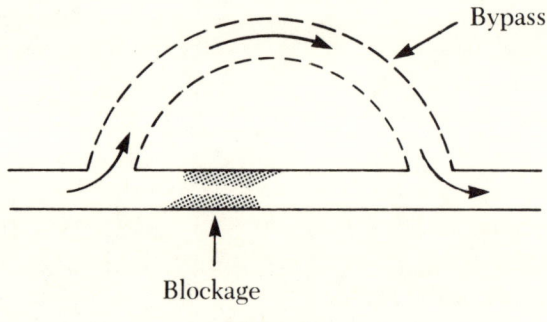

Figure 5.

Yet recently, the bypass operation has come under fire. Critics contend that many such operations are done unnecessarily: apparently physicians have been too quick to seize upon the CABG as a cure-all, when scientific evidence indicates that many patients do equally well with medication and a Heartplan. The controversy about the bypass operation is based on the definition of the word *necessary*. Advocates of bypass surgery insist that it is necessary for some patients: those who do not respond to medication and whose symptoms can be eliminated by the surgery.

In truth, there are patients for whom the bypass operation is the best therapy, and there are others for whom it is not. Let's examine the evidence.

Many patients have no symptoms and still end up having the bypass operation. Typical is the 60-year-old man whose doctor detects a slight abnormality on a routine electrocardiogram. An exercise stress test confirms the trouble. Coronary angiography shows partial blockage of two coronary arteries and a normal heart muscle. The operation is recommended because *if* an artery becomes completely blocked, the patient *may* suffer a heart attack or may die. This seems reasonable since in many patients, the first symptom of severe trouble is a heart attack or sudden death.

The patient has the bypass operation, after which he considers himself lucky to be alive. Friends who see him jogging six months later marvel at the sight, since only a while ago, he was at death's door—so they think. Unfortunately, not a shred of scientific evidence supports the contention that *this* patient will live longer because of the operation.

> During a routine physical examination, Lloyd Foster, a 62-year-old man, was discovered to have a slight abnormality on his electrocardiogram. This was confirmed by an exercise stress test, and coronary angiography showed all three of his coronary arteries were severely narrowed (more than 70 percent narrowing), but his heart muscle was absolutely normal. A coronary bypass operation was recommended.
> Mr. Foster refused the operation, saying he felt fine. He returned to work at his son-in-law's construction company.
> Four years later, Mr. Foster is still working at the age of 66. He carries heavy tools and equipment, and is still symptom-free. Repeat coronary angiography shows that two of his coronary arteries are completely closed, but his heart muscle is still normal. He developed excellent collateral circulation and did not have a heart attack. His heart is adequately supplied with oxygen and functions normally.

Many physicians now question whether patients such as Mr. Foster should have the bypass operation; the evidence suggests that they should not. Surgery is not indicated for most patients who have no symptoms. However, a risk-factor control program is essential to prevent progression of the disease and to prevent blockage that could cause a heart attack or bring about angina pectoris.

For two groups of heart patients, the bypass operation clearly does prolong life and is the best therapy: (1) patients who have severe obstruction of the left main coronary artery and (2) those with obstruction of all three major coronary arteries and a weakened heart muscle. Studies show that bypass surgery prolongs life for these patients, whether or not angina pectoris symptoms are present.

What chance do you take if you have angina or have had a heart attack, and you don't want bypass surgery? If you don't fall into one of the two groups described, your prognosis for long-term survival is as good with medical therapy as with surgery. You must weigh the risks and benefits of each form of treatment.

Who Needs a Bypass Operation?

The main indication for the bypass operation is persistent symptoms after a good try at medical therapy. A small group of patients have such severe blockage in their coronary arteries (determined by cardiac catheterization) that their risk of sudden death is high. These people are better off with the bypass operation, even if they have no symptoms, since the first major symptom for such people can be a massive heart attack or sudden death.

Whether surgery is unnecessary depends on your definition of necessity. Claims about unnecessary surgery focus on the fact that the operation does not really prolong life. This is often true. But living with chest pain every time you exert yourself is not really living, and surgery usually eliminates all cardiac symptoms, allowing patients to return to work and to active, vigorous lives. Surgical treatment also avoids the need for medications, which often have annoying and, sometimes, dangerous side-effects.

By no means do we think that everybody with coronary artery disease should have an operation, but surgery is indicated when symptoms interfere with a full life. The risk of bypass surgery in a good medical center is very low—major complications occur in only about 1 out of 100 patients—if a patient has no other serious illness.

Within the past year, the technique of coronary angioplasty has been perfected. *Angioplasty* comes from two other words: *angio*, meaning blood vessel, and *plasty*, meaning to reshape. Simpler and less traumatic than surgery, angioplasty unblocks a clogged coronary artery. The procedure can only be used for certain kinds of artery blockages, and it doesn't always work. However, it isn't a major operation, and it is often worth a try.

Technically, angioplasty is similar to cardiac catheterization, which uses a catheter with an inflatable balloon at its tip. The balloon is positioned within the coronary artery at the site of the blockage. It is then inflated with high pressure, and the blockage is pushed out of the way and broken up. The balloon is then deflated and withdrawn, leaving the coronary artery widened.

Because it is less traumatic than bypass surgery, coronary angioplasty may become the treatment of choice for patients with milder forms of coronary artery disease who don't respond well to medical therapy. It is also useful for very old or sick patients for whom the risk of surgery is unacceptably high. Today, four out of five patients experience an initial relief of symptoms with angioplasty. One out of three patients whose symptoms are relieved will have a recurrence of symptoms within a year or two. The other patients remain well for at least several years.

Many cardiologists now believe that cardiac patients who have neither left main artery disease nor three-vessel involvement with impaired heart muscle should try angioplasty if medical therapy doesn't work well.

The following are some comparisons between coronary angioplasty and the coronary artery bypass graft:

- Angioplasty is best suited for milder coronary artery disease when medical treatment fails; bypass surgery is best in severe left main coronary artery disease or in three-vessel disease where there is weakened heart muscle.
- In about one-third of cases, the coronary artery can reclose within one year after angioplasty. If the angioplasty lasts one year, the outlook is good. With bypass surgery, the same forces that were working on the coronary arteries now work on the graft, and it may eventually narrow because of progressive atherosclerosis.
- Unlike bypass surgery, angioplasty can be done again and again, with little additional risk.
- Angioplasty is less traumatic and less expensive than surgery.
- Patients whose bypass grafts eventually become occluded may be good candidates for angioplasty.

- Patients who have angioplasty may worry that the reshaped blood vessel will close resulting in a heart attack or sudden death.
- About 3 percent of patients who have had angioplasty require a bypass operation because a complication occurs during the angioplasty procedure.
- Neither angioplasty nor bypass surgery cure the underlying problem of atherosclerosis; they merely undo the effects of coronary artery narrowing. In a sense, they buy the patient additional time.

Nearly 50,000 coronary angioplasties were done in 1984. As technology is refined and expertise becomes widely available, the results of angioplasty will improve, relieving more patients of their symptoms at a lower risk.

Which Treatment Is Best for You?

If you have angina pectoris, have had a heart attack, or if angiography indicates you have coronary artery narrowing, which treatment is best suited for you—medical therapy, angioplasty, or the bypass operation?

There are no hard-and-fast answers, since your treatment depends on a variety of factors, including:

- The severity of your disease and whether your coronary vessels can be bypassed
- The duration of your symptoms
- Your medical condition, your age, and the extent to which your condition responds to medication
- The side-effects of your medication
- Whether you have already had a bypass operation and the risks you may run by having additional surgery
- Your emotional reaction to surgery

Surgery is a major ordeal requiring about ten days of hospitalization and two to three months for complete recovery. Both major and minor complications are possible. However, you will almost certainly be free of angina symptoms without large doses of medication. Also, the long-term prognosis (once you've survived the operation) is much better than with no treatment at all. Many studies have shown that once the risk of operative complications has passed, the five-year survival rates for bypass surgery are the same as age-matched control populations who have never had heart disease.

In most patients, prognosis with medical therapy (which includes a strict diet, no smoking, and reducing stress and other life-style mistakes) is about the same as with surgery. Medical therapy is certainly less traumatic and cheaper. Angina symptoms can usually be completely controlled, but some patients may require large doses of medication, and side-effects of the drugs can be a problem. Thus although the long-term outlook is similar with surgery or medicine, the surgical patient encounters most of the risk of dying at the time of the operation. For medical patients, the risk continues for a long time—this can be emotionally burdensome.

Every patient should be well-informed about the risks and benefits of all forms of therapy. Ultimately, you must choose what is best for your life-style, your condition, and your psyche. A good relationship with a physician who gets to know you, your family, your work, your life-style, and your preferences is essential.

Take as much time with your doctor as you need to get all the information you need to make a decision. Bypass surgery is usually not emergency surgery; you have time to become informed about your treatment options. Remember, they are *your* options, and the ultimate choice of treatment rests largely with you.

Some physicians have a procedural bias for or against one treatment or another. Make sure that your physician carefully assesses the need for bypass surgery and considers angioplasty or medical therapy first. Remember too that in some cases the operation clearly prolongs patients' lives, and sometimes only bypass surgery will adequately control symptoms.

If, after speaking with your doctor about your treatment options, you are still undecided, get another physician's opinion. Some patients find requesting a second opinion difficult. They feel that asking for a referral to another doctor or reserving the right to decide about a procedure somehow questions the first doctor's professionalism or credentials. However, second opinions have become a standard part of medical practice in recent years, especially when a patient is considering treatment for a serious condition. Most insurance plans today pay for and encourage second opinions.

If you have any doubts or questions about your proposed treatment, get another opinion. After all, it's your heart, your body, and your life.

Emotional Aspects of Heart Surgery

All surgery carries with it fears and worries, especially fear of being put to sleep and of being cut open. Cardiac surgery heightens these concerns because, as we have said, people often consider the heart as the very center of a person.

Patients being evaluated for heart surgery face a strange conflict. They are examined by a cardiovascular surgical team, undergoing angiography and various other medical and laboratory tests. Through all the tedium and fear, patients anxiously await a verdict about their suitability for surgery, hoping that the doctors will determine that they are good candidates. Once the case is accepted, the operation becomes a reality for the patient, who suddenly both desires and dreads the surgery.

The surgical experience itself has an enormous impact. Discuss both the anesthesia and operation with members of your surgical team. The more you know, the less subject you will be to distortion, fantasy, and anxiety about the surgery. You should have many questions about the operation. Answers will depend on the specifics of your condition and the exact surgery you require.

The heart-lung machine used in cardiac surgery is a technological marvel that serves as both heart and lungs during surgery. It removes carbon dioxide from the blood and supplies it with fresh oxygen, pumping the blood throughout the entire body.

Awakening in the recovery room can be a difficult and uncomfortable experience for any patient. Tubes, drains, intravenous infusions, nurses, and doctors are everywhere. Some patients later report that the 48-hour period immediately following surgery was the most stressful because the recovery area has an emergency room atmosphere. Most patients are heavily sedated during this time and don't remember anything.

The recovery period following surgery may take many weeks at home. Weakness and fatigue are common for up to eight weeks after the operation. Some patients feel that they have been surgically rescued; some experience a postoperative depression. For some, the realization that they have gone through surgery and must now readapt to their previous situations can be very unsettling. Some patients actually feel that they have "lost" their heart disease and find the burdens of reassuming financial and marital responsibilities upsetting. However, most patients, no matter how long they've been troubled by symptoms, readjust after surgery and feel ready to resume productive lives.

People with heart disease who successfully negotiate cardiac surgery often make an enormous emotional transition—suddenly their lives are more precious and meaningful. They reassess themselves and their priorities and often decide to alter certain life-style mistakes. The entire process, from the moment of the diagnosis to the completion of the recuperation after surgery, can be an awe-inspiring experience that provides positive physical results and inspires emotional growth.

Heart Transplants

In October 1984, the world was stunned when an anonymous infant—called Baby Fae by the press—received the heart of a baby baboon. She was born with a malformed heart that could not keep her alive, and her life was prolonged for weeks by this history-making effort. Baby Fae was the only human being to live more than one week with an animal-heart transplant.

Only a handful of animal-to-human heart transplants have ever been attempted, and all have failed. Cross-species transplants seem beyond medicine's present knowledge, but someday attempts such as Baby Fae's operation at Loma Linda, California, may succeed. The main reason some physicians are concentrating on xenografts (transplants between distantly related species) is that human donor organs are in short supply. Recent success with cyclosporine, a drug that has virtually revolutionized the transplant field, has spurred physicians to pursue xenografts. Conventional drugs used to prevent tissue rejection suppress the entire immune response system, leaving the patient vulnerable to frequent, serious infections. Cyclosporine attacks only the cells involved in tissue rejection, leaving the immune system's infection-fighting cells intact to battle bacteria and viruses.

Compatibility for cross-species transplantation is determined by three main factors: tissue type, blood group, and cellular reactions. The better these three factors match, the greater the chance that an organ transplanted from one species will be accepted by the tissues of another.

Although xenograft techniques have not been perfected, physicians hope that revolutionary changes to the transplantation field are in the near future. Then doctors may actually cross the species barrier, successfully putting animals' organs to work for man.

Human Heart Transplants

Transplanting a human heart from a suitable donor to a seriously disabled patient with end-stage failure of the heart muscle can be dramatic and successful therapy. Major improvements in therapy now prevent the body from rejecting a transplanted heart. In the best surgical centers, the three-year survival rate following cardiac transplantation is 70 percent, and most patients who survive eventually resume normal activities.

> Edward Davis had a good job and loved to participate in sports. At the age of 40 he developed severe heart muscle failure. Over a period of several months, he became increasingly short of breath, and finally could not walk even a short distance. No longer able to work, he grew progressively weaker. Complete cardiac evaluation showed an irreversible cardiomyopathy (disease of the heart muscle) with severe heart failure that did not improve with medication.
>
> A cardiac transplant operation was done, and Mr. Davis recovered well. Gradually resuming normal activities, he returned to his former job and slowly began playing his favorite sport—racquetball. Eventually, he increased the frequency and duration of his activities, and he now plays racquetball three times each week, works, and leads a full life. Without the transplant, he would have been unable to do virtually anything

but walk a very short distance, and no doubt would have died in a few months.

The Artificial Heart

Although an organized quest for a workable artificial heart began in 1963, most Americans first learned about this device in December 1982, when one was implanted into the body of Dr. Barney Clark at the University of Utah Medical School. The surgical team was headed by Dr. William DeVries, who has since performed the operation at the Humana Medical Center in Louisville, Kentucky, on a few other patients.

The Jarvik 7, the artificial heart used, is a fully implantable device that bioengineers believe will interact safely with blood. For now, scientists seem to have abandoned the search for an implantable power source along with the heart, and patients with artificial hearts are attached to an external portable power console that is cumbersome and restrictive.

It is too early to evaluate the results of the few artificial hearts implanted so far. Experiments have shown that calves can live up to ten months with an artificial heart, but the implantation of an artificial heart is experimental at present, and should be reserved for a select few patients who are willing to be research subjects to assist in the project's development. Some of the questions that need to be answered include:

- Will the material of the artificial heart damage blood cells that enter its chambers?
- Will the body "recognize" the artificial heart as a foreign substance and induce inflammation and infection?
- Will an implantable power source be developed?
- How will patients react emotionally to living "hooked up" to a machine?

Critics of the artificial heart program decry the enormous cost of this operation. Even with the surgeons' waiving fees, Dr. Clark's operation cost over $250,000, and development of a large-scale workable artificial heart program is unlikely. Our society is now focusing on reducing the cost of medical care, and continued financial support for such research may not materialize. Lack of subsidy may raise ethical issues concerning a procedure that can be performed only on those able to pay for it. Many physicians believe that the enormous sums of money involved could be better spent on preventive medicine, even though technological breakthroughs are more dramatic than eating sensibly, exercising, reducing stresses, and avoiding cigarettes. Right now, a truly effective antismoking campaign would save thousands of lives—many more than a good artificial heart.

Research on artificial heart implants will no doubt continue. For the time being, this dramatic and awe-inspiring procedure is not a practical solution for any patient who must deal with and conquer coronary artery or coronary heart disease.

11
The Future

We hope a future edition of this book will require a rewrite because of the enormous strides made in understanding heart disease, its prevention, its early diagnosis, and its treatment. This chapter speculates about what advances will most likely occur within the next few years.

Advances in Understanding the Disease

A number of crucial mechanisms must be more fully understood before physicians have a complete working model of coronary artery disease. A deeper understanding of the basic process of atherosclerosis could contribute to practical solutions to the problems of prevention, early detection, and treatment of coronary heart disease. For instance, physicians are getting closer to deciphering the cellular mechanisms that allow atherosclerotic plaque to form on the interior linings of arteries. Why does this process occur more rapidly in some people than in others? How is it speeded up or slowed down? What biological and environmental factors affect the process and can they be modified? Why do atherosclerotic changes occur in some arteries more frequently than in others? Does plaque form the same way in the coronary artery as it does in an artery of the brain? If not, how and why does the process differ? Can atherosclerosis be reversed in arteries with extensive plaque and severe narrowing? Perhaps the most important unanswered question is: What precipitates the acute symptoms such as a heart attack or sudden death in patients with known coronary disease?

All these questions and others are under intense investigation. Research scientists are close to achieving a better understanding of the disease process. Successful research could lead to dramatic advances in the prevention, diagnosis, and treatment of heart disease.

Advances in Prevention

Prevention of *any* disease is preferable to treatment, and some developments in the prevention of heart disease hold promise. For example, controlling diet, stress, and the intake of cigarettes is now considered crucial in the prevention of coronary heart disease. Some years ago, physicians maintained some doubt about the importance of these factors, but responsible physicians now think that increasing awareness of these simple preventive measures will allow people to live longer and healthier lives. As a matter of fact, most of our cardiologist friends are very careful about their diets, exercise regularly, don't smoke cigarettes, and make major efforts to deal with stresses appropriately.

Genetic factors that make certain people more vulnerable to atherosclerosis may soon be isolated. If a simple blood test could identify genetically susceptible people, these disease-prone people would have an incentive to begin prevention programs (involving proper diet, exercise, etc.) at a younger age. Early prevention could help thousands of people to avoid the ravages of atherosclerosis, heart disease, and stroke.

Advances in Diagnosis

The next best thing to preventing a disease is diagnosing it before severe symptoms or disability develop. Recent diagnostic advances use Computerized Axial Tomography (CAT) scans and improvements in angiography to allow more accurate and detailed views of the heart and its blood supply to be obtained.

Nuclear magnetic resonance (NMR) promises to be the most revolutionary detection method available to physicians. This technique is noninvasive (meaning that no tubes are inserted into the body) and does not use any form of radiation. A magnetic field is formed around the patient's body, and computer analysis produces pictures of the internal workings of the body by interpreting how various body tissues interact with the electromagnetic field.

This technique can accurately discriminate between normal cells and those that differ even slightly. The smallest atherosclerotic plaque (or the changes in the arterial wall that precede actual plaque formation) can be scrutinized. The computer's representation is a segmentalized picture, something like viewing a loaf of bread by slicing through it at various points.

In theory, a patient who is discovered to have the beginnings of atherosclerosis can be started on preventive measures long before the onset of symptomatic disease. This could result in a much lower incidence of coronary artery and coronary heart disease.

Right now, NMR is being used in a few pilot programs and is not yet available as a detection tool. It is hoped that more time and knowledge will perfect the technique and lower its cost, thus making available the most powerful diagnostic tool physicians have ever had. NMR may revolutionize medicine.

Advances in Treatment

Medical therapy is improving in many ways. New and potent variations of presently available medications are being developed. This could mean more powerful beta blockers and calcium blockers, drugs that exert their effects more specifically, with lower doses and fewer side-effects.

A whole new class of cholesterol-lowering medications that work effectively at minimal doses may be developed. We can hope for medications that shrink already-established atherosclerotic plaques, causing atherosclerotic lesions to regress and leaving the arteries wide open and unobstructed!

One area of recent interest is the use of anticoagulants such as streptokinase. When injected into the bloodstream of a patient who is having a heart attack due to thrombosis of an artery, streptokinase dissolves the artery-blocking clot. The therapy's main drawback is that the streptokinase must be injected very soon after the clot forms to be effective. There is also a risk of severe bleeding. But this treatment may be a model for an entirely new class of medications that can dissolve clots and cause plaque regression or even prevent the formation of atherosclerotic plaques! At present, some medical centers are using streptokinase in conjunction with angioplasty as therapy for heart attacks.

Studies have begun with tissue plasminogen activator (TPA), which attaches to the clot in the coronary artery and helps dissolve it. The advantage of this technique is that TPA does not cause bleeding from other areas of the body. High-risk patients may someday carry around a syringe of TPA with which to inject themselves at the first sign of a heart attack.

Surgical therapy will continue to improve in the next few years. For instance, current data indicate that using the internal mammary artery as graft material instead of a saphenous vein greatly improves the long-term survival of the graft. Improvements in surgical techniques, anesthesia, and the heart-lung machine will lower the risks of surgery and the rate of serious complications. Similarly, coronary angioplasty in conjunction with medical therapy (such as streptokinase and other to-be-developed drugs) may be refined and used more widely.

Despite debate about the desirability of cross-species transplants, they will probably continue as an area of intensive investigation. As more is understood about the phenomenon of tissue rejection, xenografts may become more feasible. Right now, certain parts of other mammals' internal organs are used for "spare parts" in various operations, including heart valves supplied by pigs and cows. A solution to the problem of tissue rejection may expand this field fantastically.

Any development in one area—prevention, diagnosis, or treatment—often has important repercussions in other areas. For instance, development of a simple test to pinpoint disease-prone individuals will have an enormous impact on prevention and medical therapy, since convincing people to reduce their risks is much easier if they know their risk is very high. If developed, medications that will prevent the deposit of artery-clogging materials can then be used for the disease-prone people targeted by the screening test.

A Word of Caution

As with other areas of medicine, the future seems very bright. Basic research and clinical medicine will most likely merge their findings to herald a new era in the understanding, diagnosis, and treatment of coronary artery and coronary heart disease. Our children will probably have a very different perspective of this disease.

We urge one word of caution. Sometimes we become too enthusiastic about the marvels of scientific innovation. We often think that sophisticated technology will solve all our problems, but, although it may help in certain crucial areas, such wizardry isn't the answer to everything. We must beware of innovations that look like panaceas but are really empty promises.

At this moment, despite all scientific advances, one undeniable truth remains: The battle against heart disease can be most successfully waged by as simple a concept as *prevention*. Sensible eating and exercising habits, reducing unnecessary stresses, and avoiding smoking can do more right now than the latest billion-dollar gadgetry and all the technological contraptions in the world.

We must know our own bodies and be aware of what harms or helps them. We must take responsibility for our own health and play an active role in maintaining our own well-being.

You owe it to yourself to develop and live your very own Heartplan.

Selected References

Adsetti, C. A., and J. G. Bruhn: "Short-term Group Psychotherapy for Post-Myocardial Infarction Patients and Their Wives," *Canadian Medical Association Journal*, **99**: 557-584 (1968).

Arntzenius, Alexander, C., et al.: "Diet, Lipoproteins, and the Progression of Coronary Atherosclerosis," *New England Journal of Medicine*, **312**: 805-810 (March 1985).

Baer, L., and I. Radichevich: "Cigarette Smoking in Hypertensive Patients," *American Journal of Medicine*, **78**: 564-568 (April 1985).

Benson, H.: *The Relaxation Response*, Morrow, New York, 1975.

Bernstein, Barton J.: "The Artificial Heart: A Study in Myopia," *MD Magazine*, (September 1984).

Braunwald, E.: "Coronary Artery Spasm as a Cause of Myocardial Ischemia," *Journal of Laboratory Clinical Medicine*, **97**: 299-312 (1981).

Brown, V., H. Ginsberg, and W. Kamally: "Diet and the Decrease of Coronary Heart Disease," *American Journal of Cardiology*, **54** (1984).

Bruhn, J. G., B. Chandler, and S. Wolf: "A Psychological Study of Survivors and Non-Survivors of Myocardial Infarction," *Psychosomatic Medicine*, **31**: 1-19 (1969).

Cannon, W.: "Voodoo Death," *American Anthropologist*, **44**: 169-181 (1942).

Case, R. B., et al.: "Type A Behavior and Survival after Acute Myocardial Infarction," *New England Journal of Medicine*, **312**: 737-741 (March 1985).

Castelli, W. P.: "The Epidemiology of Coronary Heart Disease, The Framingham Study," *Journal of the American Medical Association*, **76**: 4-12 (1984).

Cousins, N.: "Anatomy of an Illness (as Perceived by the Patient)," *New England Journal of Medicine*, **295**: 1458-1463 (1976).

———: *The Healing Heart: Antidotes to Panic and Helplessness*, Norton, New York, 1983.

Dimsdale, J.: "Emotional Causes of Sudden Death," *American Journal of Psychiatry*, **134**: 1361-1366 (1977).

Eliot, Robert S.: *Stress and the Heart*, Futura, Mount Kisco, N.Y., 1974.

———, and A. D. Forker: "Emotional Stress and Cardiac Disease," *Journal of the American Medical Association*, **237**: 2325-2326 (1976).

Engel, G. L.: "Psychologic Stress: Vasodepressor (Vasovagal) Syncope, and Sudden Death," *Annals of Internal Medicine*, **89**: 403-412 (1978).

———: "Sudden and Rapid Death During Psychologic Stress: Folklore or Folk Wisdom?" *Annals of Internal Medicine*, **74**: 771-782 (1971).

———: *Psychological Development in Health and Disease*, Saunders, Philadelphia, 1962.

Enos, W., and R. Holmes: "Coronary Disease among United States Soldiers Killed in Action in Korea," *Journal of the American Medical Association*, **152**: 1090-1093 (1953).

Friedman, M., et al.: "Feasibility of Altering Type A Behavior Pattern after Myocardial Infarction," *Circulation*, **66**: 83-92 (1982).

———, and R. H. Rosenman: *Type A Behavior and Your Heart*, Fawcett Columbia Books, New York, 1974.

———, ———, and V. Corall: "Changes in the Serum Cholesterol and Blood Clotting Time in Men Subjected to Cyclic Variation of Occupational Stress," *Circulation*, **17**: 852-861 (1958).

Gentry, W. D., and R. B. Williams: *Psychological Aspects of Myocardial Infarction and Coronary Care*, Mosby, St. Louis, 1975.

Hellstrom, H. R.: "Coronary Artery Vasospasm: The Likely Immediate Cause of Acute Myocardial Infarction," *British Heart Journal*, **41**: 426-432 (1979).

Helsing, K. J., and M. Szeklo: "Mortality after Bereavement," *American Journal of Epidemiology*, **114**: 41-52 (1981).

Hjermann, I., et al.: "Effect of Diet and Smoking Intervention on the Incidence of Coronary Heart Disease," *Lancet*, **2**: 1303-1310 (1981).

Holmes, T. H., and R. H. Rahe: "The Social Readjustment Rating Scale," *Journal of Psychosomatic Research*, **2**: 213 (1967).

Jenkins, C. D.: "Recent Evidence Supporting Psychologic Social Risk Factors for Coronary Disease," *New England Journal of Medicine*, **294**: 987-994, 1033-1038 (1976).

Kannel, W. B., et al.: "Epidemiological Assessment of the Role of Physical Activity and Fitness in Development of Cardiovascular Disease," *American Heart Journal*, **109**: 876-885 (April 1985).

Kaplan, Norman M.: "Non-Drug Treatment of Hypertension," *Annals of Internal Medicine*, **102**: 359-373 (1985).

Killip, T.: "Coronary Bypass Surgery: Where We Stand Today," *Drug Therapy*, (October 1984).

Kones, R. J.: "Emotional Stress, Plasma Catecholamines, Cardiac Risk Factors, and Atherosclerosis," *Angiology*, **30**: 327-336 (1979).

Kushi, L. H., et al.: "Diet and 20 Year Mortality from Coronary Heart Disease," *New England Journal of Medicine*, **312**(13): 811-818 (March 1985).

Lynch, J., et al.: "The Effects of Human Contact in Coronary Care Patients," *Journal of Nervous and Mental Diseases*, **158**: 88-99 (1974).

McLane, M., H. Krop, and J. Mehta: "Psychosexual Adjustment and Counseling after Myocardial Infarction," *Annals of Internal Medicine*, **92**: 514-519 (1980).

Marx, J. L.: "Coronary Artery Spasms and Heart Disease, *Science*, **208**: 1227-1230 (1980).

Maseri, A., et al.: "Coronary Vasospasm as a Possible Cause of Myocardial Infarction," *New England Journal of Medicine*, **299**: 1271-1277 (1978).

Massie, E., et al.: "Sudden Death During Coitus: Fact or Fiction?" *Medical Aspects of Human Sexuality*, **3**: 22-26 (1969).

Moore, K., M. Folk-Lightz, and M. J. Nolen: "The Joy of Sex after a Heart Attack: Counseling the Cardiac Patient," *Nursing*, **7**: 53-55 (1977).

Moss, A., and B. Wyner: "Tachycardia in House Officers Presenting Cases at Grand Rounds," *Annals of Internal Medicine*, **72**: 255-256 (1970).

Myers, A., and H. A. Dewar: "Circumstances Attending 100 Sudden Deaths from Coronary Artery Disease with Coroner's Necropsies," *British Heart Journal*, **37**: 1133-1143 (1975).

Parkes, C. M., B. Benjamin, and R. G. Fitzgerald: "Broken Heart: A Statistical Study of Increased Mortality among Widowers," *British Medical Journal*, **1**: 740-743 (1969).

Preston, T. A.: "Bypass Surgery: A Placebo?" *MD Magazine* (February 1985).

Rahe, R. H.: "Stress and Strain in Coronary Heart Disease," *Journal of the South Carolina Medical Association*, **72**: 7-14 (1976).

———, et al.: "A Model for Life Changes and Illness Research," *Archives of General Psychiatry*, **31**: 172-177 (1974).

———, and E. Lind: "Psychosocial Factors and Sudden Cardiac Death: A Pilot Study," *Journal of Psychosomatic Research*, **15**: 19-24 (1971).

———, and M. Romo: "Recent Life Changes and the Onset of Myocardial Infarction and Sudden Death in Helsinki," in E. K. Gunderson and R. Rahe (eds.), *Life Stress and Illness*, Charles C. Thomas, Springfield, Ill., 1974, pp. 105-120.

——, M. Romo, L. Bennet, et al.: "Recent Life Changes Preceding Myocardial Infarction and Abrupt Coronary Death," *Archives of Internal Medicine*, **133**: 221-228 (1974).

——, H. W. Ward, and V. Hayes: "Brief Group Therapy in Myocardial Infarction Rehabilitation: Three-to-Four-Year Follow Up of a Controlled Trial," *Psychosomatic Medicine*, **41**: 229-242 (1979).

Reich, P., et al.: "Acute Psychological Disturbances Preceding Life-Threatening Ventricular Arrhythmias," *Journal of the American Medical Association*, **246**: 233-235 (1981).

Rifkind, B.: "Lipid Research Clinics Coronary Primary Prevention Trail: Results and Implications," *American Journal of Cardiology*, **54** (1984).

Rosenman, R. H., and M. Friedman: "Modifying Type A Behavior Pattern," *Journal of Psychosomatic Research*, **21**: 323-331 (1977).

——, and ——: "Neurogenic Factors in Pathogenesis of Coronary Heart Disease," *Medical Clinics of North America*, **58**: 269-279, (1974).

Ruberman, W., et al.: "Education, Psychosocial Stress and Sudden Cardiac Death," *Journal of Chronic Diseases*, **36**: 151-160 (1983).

Schatzkin, A., et al.: "The Epidemiology of Sudden Unexpected Death: Risk Factors for Men and Women in the Framingham Heart Study," *American Heart Journal*, **107** (1984).

Schiffer, F., et al.: "The Quiz Electrocardiogram: A New Diagnostic and Research Technique for Evaluating a Relation Between Emotional Stress and Ischemic Heart Disease," *American Journal of Cardiology*, **37**: 41-47 (1976).

Schonfeld, G., J. Witztum, and P. Basich: "Effect of Dietary Cholesterol and Fatty Acids on Plasma Lipoproteins," *Journal of Clinical Investigation*, **69**: 1072-1080 (1982).

Selye, H.: *The Stress of Life*, McGraw-Hill, New York, 1956.

Slone, D., et al.: "Relation of Cigarette Smoking to Myocardial Infarction in Young Women," *New England Journal of Medicine*, **298**: 1273 (1978).

Swinn, R. M., L. Brock, and C. A. Edie: "Behavior Therapy for Type A Patients," *American Journal of Cardiology*, **36**: 269 (1975).

Taggert, P., D. Gibbons, and W. Somerville: "Some Effects of Motor Car Driving on the Normal and Abnormal Heart," *British Medical Journal*, **4**: 130-134 (1969).

Thomas, C. B., and R. L. Greenstreet: "Psychobiological Characteristics in Youth as Predictors of Five Disease States: Suicide, Mental Illness, Hypertension, Coronary Heart Disease and Tumor," *Johns Hopkins Medical Journal*, **132**: 16-43 (1973).

Trimble, G. X.: "The Coital Coronary," *Medical Aspects of Human Sexuality*, **4**: 64-72 (1970).

Underwood, D. A.: "Symptomatic Coronary Artery Disease in Patients Aged 21 to 30 Years," *American Journal of Cardiology*, **55**: 631-634 (March 1985).

Weiss, T., B. Engel, and J. Beyer: "Operant Conditioning of Heart Rate in Patients with PVC's," *Psychosomatic Medicine*, **33**: 301-321 (1971).

Wishnie, H. A., T. P. Hackett, and N. H. Cassem: "Psychological Hazards of Convalescence Following Myocardial Infarction," *Journal of the American Medical Association*, **215**: 1292-1296 (1971).

Wolf, S.: "Psychosocial Forces in Myocardial Infarction and Sudden Death," in L. Levi (ed.), *Society, Stress and Disease*, vol. 1, Oxford Press, New York, 1971, pp. 324-330.

Index

About Your Heart and Smoking (American Heart Association), 156
Adrenal glands, 32
Adrenaline, 32, 33, 145
Aerobic exercise, 138–145
  aerobic dancing, 144
  bicycling, 144, 174
  cool-down period after, 139
  jogging and running, 141–143, 174
  swimming, 143, 144, 174
  walking, 143, 174
  warm-up before, 138–139
  (*See also* Exercise; Exercise programs)
Age and aging:
  and blood pressure, 17
  and risk of cardiovascular disease, 15
  and risk of fatal heart attacks, 15
  and selection of exercise programs, 11, 139, 143
  and target zone, 139, 140
Air pollution, 143

Air travel, 99, 115
Alcohol consumption, 19, 29, 114–115
Aldactone, 161
Aldomet, 161
Altered states of consciousness, 146–149
American Cancer Society, 154
American Heart Association, 19, 22, 101, 115, 137–138, 166
  RISKO heart-hazard appraisal questionnaire of, 23–26
  stop-smoking program of, 155, 156
American Heart Association Cookbook (Eishelman and Winston, eds.), 136
American Lung Association, stop-smoking program of, 155
Ammonia, 28
Anesthesia, 190, 198
Angina pectoris, 9, 10, 177
  from chronic stress, 94–95
  cigarette smoking and, 149–152
  drug therapy for, 80, 160

Angina pectoris *(cont.)*:
  and risk of further cardiovascular disease, 16
  and sexual activity, 169-172, 175
  surgical treatment of, 183-194
Angiography, coronary, 12, 22, 49, 62, 184, 185
Angioplasty (*see* Coronary angioplasty)
Anxiety:
  after heart attack, 62-64
  reduction of, in CCU, 58-59
  about sexual activity, 169-172, 175
Aorta, 5, 8, 183
Appliance repairs, 99
Appointments:
  medical and dental, 98, 177
  with service and trades workers, 99
Apresoline, 161
Arrhythmias, 6, 9, 13, 19, 32, 55-58
Arteries, 5-6
  aortic, 5, 8, 183
  radial, 6
  (*See also* Atherosclerosis; Coronary arteries; Coronary artery disease)
Artificial hearts, 193-194
Ashe, Arthur, 177
Aspirin, 29
Atherosclerosis, 7-8
  cigarette smoking and, 8
  coronary artery disease resulting from, 7-9, 31, 141
  diabetics at risk for, 16
  dietary cholesterol and, 8
  drug therapy for, 197, 198
  exercise and, 138
  hypertension and, 8, 17
  and risk of cardiovascular disease, 16
  slow development of, 7-8, 10
  stress and, 8
Athletes:
  coronary artery disease in, 141-142
  HDL levels in, 19
Ativan, 162
Automatic teller machines, 96

Banks, minor irritants at, 96-97
Baylor University, 138
Benson, Herbert, 146, 148
Beta blockers, 159, 160
Beverages, 102-103
  alcoholic, 19, 29, 114-115
  coffee, 28-29, 102, 114
Bicycling, 144, 174
Biofeedback, 148-149
Birth control pills, 20, 25, 28
Blood:
  in heart-lung machine, 190, 198
  oxygen in, 5-6, 19, 190
  transport of, 5-6
Blood clots (thrombi), arterial, 9, 10
  drug therapy for, 198
  fight-or-flight response and, 32, 40
  oral contraceptives and, 20
Blood pressure, 6
  diastolic, 6
  emotional stress and, 27-28, 32, 33, 36, 145
  high (*see* Hypertension)
  measurement of, 6, 17, 27-28
  nicotine and, 19
  normal values for, 17
  oral contraceptives and, 20
  relaxation response and, 149
  systolic, 6, 24, 25
Blood vessels, 5-6
  length of, 5
  veins, 6, 183
  (*See also* Arteries; Coronary arteries; Coronary artery disease)
Boston University Medical Center, 17
Bowling, 145
Brain, oxygen in, 55
Breakfast, 102
  suggested menus for, 116-130
Breathlessness (dyspnea), 160, 161
British Medical Journal, 1-2
Bypass surgery (*see* Coronary bypass surgery)

Calan, 161
Calcium blockers, 161

Calling It Quits (HEW), 156
Calorie banking, 102, 116
Carbohydrate metabolism, 16
Carbohydrates, dietary, 102, 105
Carbon monoxide, 19, 28
Cardiac arrest, 55, 57
Cardiac care units (CCUs), 57-59, 163
  heart monitoring in, 57-58
  visiting patients in, 58-59
Cardiagen, 161
Cardiovascular disease:
  economic impact of, xi
  future medical advances in, 195-199
    diagnosis, 196-197
    prevention, 196
  Heartplan for (*see* Heartplan)
  risk for, 13-30
    age and, 15
    alcohol consumption and, 19, 29
    cholesterol and, 18-20, 22, 24, 25
    cigarette smoking and, 16, 19-20, 23-25, 28, 29, 150-151, 159
    coffee consumption and, 28-29
    current heart disease and, 16
    diabetes and, 16
    emotional entrapment and, 42-46, 48-49
    exercise and, 20, 23, 137-138, 141-142
    family history and, 16, 22, 27, 30, 142
    frequently asked questions about, 27-30
    gender and, 16
    hypertension and, 16, 20
    major life changes and, 49-52
    obesity and, 20, 23-25, 29
    oral contraceptives and, 20
    RISKO heart-hazard appraisal of, 23-26
    Sisyphus syndrome and, 37-42, 48-49
    stress and, 16, 21-23, 31-52
    type A behavior and, 46-49
  sexual activity and, 169-172

Cardiovascular disease *(cont.)*:
  (*See also* Atherosclerosis; Coronary artery disease; Heart attacks; Strokes)
CAT (Computerized Axial Tomography) scans, 197
Catheterization, coronary, 186
Cheese, 103
Chest pain (*see* Angina pectoris)
Chicago heart disease study, 23-26
Chicken Marsala, Heartplan, 134-135
Chili, Heartplan vegetarian, 131-132
Chinese cuisine, 113
Cholesterol, dietary, 8, 18, 19, 102, 103, 105, 106
Cholesterol, serum, 7, 18-20, 22, 24, 25
  coffee consumption and, 29
  drug therapy for reduction of, 161, 197
  emotional stress and, 33, 145
Cigarette smoking, 19-20
  as addiction, 151-153
  angina and, 149-152
  atherosclerosis and, 8
  heart rate and, 19
  life expectancy and, 20
  low-tar, 28
  quitting, 149-156
    benefits of, 20, 23, 150, 152, 153
    fighting denial in, 151
    with nicotine supplements, 156
    organized programs for, 154-155
    weight gain associated with, 152
    withdrawal symptoms from, 152-154
  and risk for cardiovascular disease, 16, 19-20, 23-25, 28, 29, 150-151, 159
  as self-destructive behavior, 151-153
  by women, 20, 25
Claiborne, Craig, 136, 177
Clark, Barney, 193
Clearing the Air (HEW), 156
Coffee consumption, 28-29, 102, 114
Coleslaw, Heartplan, 132

Collaterals, 64, 138
Commuting, 93, 97-98
Competitiveness, 46, 47, 88
Computerized Axial Tomography (CAT) scans, 197
Congestive heart failure, 6
　drug therapy for, 160, 161
Consciousness, altered states of, 146-149
Cooper, Kenneth H., 145
Corgard, 160
Coronary angiography, 12, 22, 49, 62, 184, 185
Coronary angioplasty, 186-188
　bypass surgery vs., 187-188
　candidates for, 187
Coronary arteries, 7-9
　calcium blockers and, 161
　collateral, 64, 138
　nitroglycerine and, 160
　spasms in, 32, 40, 56
Coronary artery disease:
　artificial heart implantation for, 193-194
　atherosclerosis resulting in, 7-9, 141
　bypass surgery for, 50, 62, 63, 65, 149-150, 183-190
　coronary angioplasty for, 186-188
　diagnosis of, 10-13, 196-197
　HDL as protection against, 18-19
　prevalence of, 7
　selecting best treatment for, 188-190
　three vessel involvement, 8, 187
Coronary bypass surgery, 50, 62, 63, 65, 149-150, 183-190
　candidates for, 185-190
　coronary angioplasty as alternative to, 186-188
　criticisms of, 184-186
　frequency of, 184
　risks of, 186
　technique of, 183-184
Coronary catheterization, 186
Cousins, Norman, 64-65, 78, 177
Craig Claiborne's Gourmet Diet (Claiborne and Franay), 136

Crash diets, 102
Cross-country skiing, 144-145
Cyclosporine, 191-192

Dairy products, 102, 103, 110
Dancing, aerobic, 144
Daydreaming, 90
Deadlines, 93
Deep muscle relaxation, 95
Deliveries, scheduling of, 99
Dental appointments, 98
Depression, 63, 80
　in family members, 180
　postoperative, 191
Desserts, 110
　in restaurants, 114
DeVries, William, 193
Diabetes:
　dietary control of, 16, 102
　and risk of cardiovascular disease, 16
Diastolic pressure, 6
Diet and nutrition:
　cholesterol in, 8, 18, 19, 102, 103, 105, 106
　diabetic, 16, 102
　family involvement in, 174, 176-177
　salt in, 17, 18, 109-110, 178
　(*See also* Heartplan--diet and nutrition in)
Digitalis, 160
Digoxin, 160
Diuretics, 161
Diuril, 161
Doctors (*see* Physicians)
Drug therapy, 159-163
　for angina, 80, 160
　aspirin, 29
　for atherosclerosis, 197, 198
　beta blockers, 159, 160
　for blood clots, 198
　calcium blockers, 161
　for congestive heart failure, 160, 161
　digitalis, 160
　diuretics, 161

Drug therapy *(cont.)*:
  after heart attack, 58, 198
  for hypertension, 18, 140, 157, 160-161
  monitoring response to, 13, 162
  nitroglycerine, 80, 160
  patient compliance with, 177
  questioning physician about, 157
  for reduction of cholesterol and triglyceride levels, 161, 197
  side effesct of, 162, 189
    sexual dysfunction, 171-172
  for stroke prevention, 29
  for tissue rejection, 191-192
  tranquilizers, 58, 161-162
Dyazide, 161
Dyspnea, 160, 161

Eastern European cuisine, 112
Eat To Win (Haas), 136
Echocardiograms, 12-13
Edema, 160, 161
Eggplant spread, Heartplan, 134
Eggs, 19, 103, 131
Eishelman, Ruthe, 136
Electricians, 99
Electrocardiograms (ECGs), 11
  in exercise stress tests, 11
  in routine physical examinations, 11, 162
Eliot, Robert, 43
Emergency rooms, 57, 163
Emotional entrapment, xii, 42-46
  invisible, 43, 82-86
  lessening of, 78-86
  obvious, 43, 79-82
  self-diagnosis questionnaire for, 44-46
  Sisyphus syndrome and type A behavior combined with, 48-49
Exercise:
  anaerobic, 138
  chest pains resulting from, 9
  HDL levels elevated by, 19, 138
  heart rate affected by, 5, 139, 140
  isometric, 138

Exercise *(cont.)*:
  and risk of cardiovascular disease, 20, 23, 137-138, 141-142
  (*See also* Aerobic exercise; Exercise programs)
Exercise and Your Heart (American Heart Association), 137-138
Exercise programs:
  aerobic, 138-145
  dos and don'ts for, 139-141
  family participation in, 174
  for heart attack recovery, 139
  hypertension controlled with, 18
  selection of:
    aging and, 11, 139, 143
    physical examination before, 11, 139, 140
Exercise stress test, 11, 141, 171, 184, 185

Fad diets, 102
Fairmont hotel chain, 115
Family members, 173-181
  depression in, 180
  guilt feelings of, 175-176
  as Heartplan particpants, 174-175
  overprotectedness by, 175, 179-180
  questions frequently asked by, 176-181
  in stress management, 174, 175
Fast-food cuisine, 110
Fatalism, 176
Fats, dietary, 102-104, 179
  cholesterol, 8, 18, 19, 102, 103, 105, 106
Favaloro, Rene, 183
Fibrillation, cardiac, 55, 56
Fight-or-flight response, 31-33, 40, 44, 48, 91, 95, 100
  defusing of, 146-149
Financial concerns, 96
Fish, 105, 106
  Heartplan baked fish, 134
  in restaurants, 111-114
Fixx, Jim, 141-142
Food & Wine Magazine, 136

Forker, Alan, 43
Four Seasons hotel chain, 115
Framingham heart disease study, 23-26, 46
Franay, Pierre, 136
Free-floating hostility, 46, 47, 88
  lessening of, 91-92
French toast, Heartplan, 130-131
Fried foods, 104, 110, 179
Friedman, Meyer, 46, 48, 87-89, 91

Games, losing at, 92
Garlic salt, 110
Gazpacho, Heartplan, 131
Gelatin, 110
Gender:
  HDL levels and, 19
  and risk of cardiovascular disease, 16
  (*See also* Women)
German cuisine, 112
German-style potato salad, Heartplan, 132
Goals, setting of, 71-78, 92
Golf, 145
Green beans, Heartplan spicy, 132-133
Grocery shopping, 97, 109
Group sessions, post-heart attack, 163-166
  emphasis in, 163, 164
  playing roles in, 164

Haas, Robert, 136
Haig, Alexander, 65, 177
Healing Heart, The (Cousins), 64-65, 78
Health, Education and Welfare Department, U.S., 18, 101, 156
Heart:
  artificial, 193-194
  collateral vessels in, 64, 138
  electrical stimulation of, 58
  electrical system of, 6, 13, 55, 56
  emotions associated with, 3

Heart *(cont.)*:
  enlargement of, 11
  fibrillation of, 55, 56
  rhythmic disturbances of, 6, 9, 13, 19, 32, 55-58
  structure of, 5
Heart attacks, 53-59
  adjustments after, 61-65
  annual number of, xi
  common concerns after, 62-65
  complications of, 57
  diagnosis of, 11, 12, 57
  drug therapy after, 58, 198
  emotional entrapment leading to, 44
  family history of, 16, 27
  fatal, 55-56
    age distribution of, 15
    cigarette smoking and, 20
    fear of, 62
    physical inactivity and, 138
    physiology of, 55
  as first symptoms of cardiovascular disease, 10, 55
  period of greatest risk after, 58
  recovery from:
    in CCU, 57-59, 163
    exercise program for, 139
    at home, 61-65
    in post-heart attack group sessions, 163-166
  return-to-work rate after, 164
  risk for:
    in athletes, 19, 141-142
    cigarette smoking and, 19-20, 159
    exercise and, 138
    gender and, 19
    HDL levels and, 19
    and modification of type A behavior, 87-88
    serum cholesterol and, 19
  self-image after, 178
  sexual activity after, 169-172, 175
  silent, 55
  Sisyphus syndrome leading to, 40
  symptoms of, 9, 53-57
  type A behavior leading to, 48, 87-88

Heart disease (*see* Cardiovascular disease)
Heart-lung machines, 190, 198
Heart monitors, 13, 57-58
Heart rate:
  cigarette smoking and, 19
  emotional stress and, 32
  exercise and, 5, 139, 140
  during intercourse, 170-171
  maximal, 139
  resting, 5
Heart transplants, 191-192, 198
Heart valves, 5
  diseased, 6, 12-13
  examination of, with echocardiograms, 12-13
Heartplan, 68-166
  diet and nutrition in, 101-137
    dining at friends' homes, 111, 179
    family involvement in, 174, 176-179
    recipes, 107-110, 130-136
    restaurant dining, 111-115, 179
    suggested menus, 115-130
  exercise in, 137-145
  family members in, 174-179
  lessening emotional entrapment in, 78-86
    invisible entrapment, 82-86
    obvious entrapment, 79-82
  medical program in, 156-166
    medical intervention, 159-163
    patient compliance with, 177
    post-heart attack group sessions, 163-166
    relationship with physician, 157-159, 162, 169-172, 189
  modifying type A behavior in, 86-92
  quitting smoking in, 149-156
  reducing stresses in, 92-101, 163-165
  reducing time urgency in, 89-91
  relaxation in, 145-149
  setting new priorities and realistic goals in, 71-78
  introspection in, 76

Heartplan *(cont.)*:
  role of material accomplishments in, 75-76
High-density lipoprotein (HDL), 18-20, 22, 29
  exercise and, 19, 138
Hilton hotel chain, 115
Holmes, Thomas H., 50
Holter monitors, 13
Hospitals:
  cardiac care units in, 57-59, 163
  emergency rooms in, 57, 163
  post-heart attack group sessions in, 163-166
  surgery in, 183-194
  trip to, 57
Hostility (*see* Free-floating hostility)
Hurry sickness, 89-91
Hydrodiuril, 161
Hydrogen cyanide, 28
Hygroton, 161
Hypertension:
  alcohol consumption and, 29
  atherosclerosis and, 8, 17
  control of, 17-18, 178-179
    with drug therapy, 18, 140, 157, 160-161
    with exercise, 18
    with weight reduction, 18, 161, 178-179
  diagnosis of, 17
  family history of, 16, 17
  prevalence of, 17
  and risk of further cardiovascular disease, 16-18, 20
  salt intake and, 17, 18, 110, 178
Hypnosis, 95, 148, 149, 155
Hypochondriasis, 63
Hypothalamus, 32

Ice milk, 110
Immune system, organ transplants and, 191-192
Inderal, 160
Indian vegetable casserole, Heartplan, 133

Insulin, 16
Internal scanning, 100
Intravenous infusions (IVs), 57
Introspection, 76
Invisible entrapment, 43
   case history of, 82-83
   feelings associated with, 83
   lessening of, 82-86
Isometric exercise, 138
Italian cuisine, 105, 112-114
IVs (intravenous infusions), 57

Japanese cuisine, 113
Jarvik 7, 193
Jobs (*see* Workplace)
Jogging, 141-143, 174
Johnson, Virginia E., 170
Journal of the American Medical Association, 43
Journey of rediscovery, 91

Kissinger, Henry, 65, 177

Lanoxin, 160
Lasix, 161
Laughter, 92, 100, 163
Librium, 162
Life changes (*see* Major life changes)
Life expectancy:
   cigarette smoking and, 20
   coronary bypass surgery and, 186
Lipoproteins, 18-19
   high density (HDL), 18-20, 22, 29, 138
Liver, cholesterol production in, 18
Loafing, 90, 145
Lopressor, 160
Losing, practicing at, 92

Major life changes, 49-52, 93
   minimizing stress from, 94
   minor irritants arising from, 96
   Social Readjustment Rating Scale and, 50-52

Marathon running, 143
Margarine, 104
Marinara sauce, Heartplan, 135-136
Mariott hotel chain, 115
Masters, William H., 170
Masturbation, 171
Material accomplishments, more personal and human rewards vs., 75-76
Meats, 102-105, 112, 116
Medicine (*see* Drug therapy)
Meditation, 95, 146-149
Menopause, and risk of cardiovascular disease, 16
Menus, suggested, 115-130
Mexican cuisine, 113-114, 131-132
Minipress, 161
Multiple gated acquisition (MUGA) scans, 12
Muscle relaxation, deep, 95
Myocardial infarctions (*see* Heart attacks)

Nautilus weight program, 145
New Aerobics, The (Cooper), 145
Nicotine, 19, 28, 156
Nitroglycerine, 80
Nuclear cardiac scans, 11-12
Nuclear magnetic resonance (NMR), 197
Nurses:
   cardiac care, 57
   rehabilitation, 163
Nutrition (*see* Diet and nutrition)

Obesity:
   hypertension and, 17, 18
   as risk for cardiovascular disease, 20, 23-25, 29
   (*See also* Weight reduction)
Obvious entrapment, 43
   case history of, 79-81
   conquering of, 79-82
Oils, cooking, 103, 104
Olive oil, 103, 104

Omelet, Heartplan, 131
Onion salt, 110
Oral contraceptives, 20, 25, 28
Oxygen:
  in blood, 5-6, 19, 190
  brain deprived of, 55
  cigarette smoking and, 19
  heart tissue deprived of, 9, 19, 55

Pancreas, 16
Panic attacks, 56
Passports, 99
Peppers, Heartplan stuffed, 132
Physicians:
  appointments with, 98, 177
  patients' relationships with, 157-159, 162, 169-172, 189
  reluctance of, to discuss sexuality, 169-170, 172
  as role models, 158
  second opinions from, 189-190
Pickles, 110
Plaque, arterial, 7-8, 10, 18, 138, 141, 197
Pollock, 106
Positive reinforcement, 90-91
Potassium depletion, 161
Potato chips, 109, 110
Potato salad, Heartplan German-style, 132
Poultry, 105, 107-109
  Heartplan chicken Marsala, 134-135
Pretzels, 109, 110
Priorities, setting of, 71-78, 91, 92
Procardia, 161
Progressive relaxation, 146
Protein, dietary, 102
Psychological counseling, 80
  as alternative to tranquilizers, 162
  for cardiac invalidism, 178
  for modification of type A behavior, 88, 89
  for sexual difficulties, 172
Pulse (see Heart rate)

Race-walking, 144
Radial arteries, 6
Rahe, Richard H., 50, 89, 163-164
Relaxation response, 146-149
Relaxation Response, The (Benson), 146
Relaxation techniques, 95, 145-149
Restaurants, 111-115, 179
  American steak houses, 112
  Chinese, 113
  desserts in, 114
  fast-food, 110
  German and Eastern European, 112
  Italian, 112-113
  Japanese, 113
  Mexican, 113-114
Rice dishes, Heartplan:
  scented rice, 134
  wild rice with mushrooms, 131
RISKO heart-hazard appraisal, 23-26
Rosenman, Ray H., 46, 87-89, 91
Running, 141-143

Salt intake, 17, 18, 109-110, 178
Saphenous veins, 183
Sashimi, 113
Scented rice, Heartplan, 134
Second opinions, 189-190
Self-reward systems, 90-91, 100
Senate Select Committee on Nutrition and Human Needs, 101
Serax, 162
Service workers, minor irritants from, 99
Seventh-Day Adventists, stop-smoking program of, 155
Sexual activity, 169-172, 175
  benefits of, 171
  drug therapy and, 171-172
Shellfish, 105, 106
Sheraton hotel chain, 115
Sherbet, 110
Shopping habits, 91
  food, 97, 109
Silent heart attacks, 55
Sisyphus syndrome, xii, 37-42

Sisyphus syndrome *(cont.)*:
  case histories of, 39-40, 71-73, 76-77
  characteristic profile of, 38-39
  emotional entrapment and type A behavior combined with, 48-49
  modification of, in post-heart attack group sessions, 164
  self-diagnosis questionnaire for, 41-42
Skiing, cross-country, 144-145
Smiling, 91-92
Smokenders, 155, 165
Smoking (*see* Cigarette smoking)
Social Readjustment Rating Scale, 50-52
Softball, 145
Soy sauce, 110, 113
Spanish cuisine, 114
Spices and herbs, 105, 109, 110, 178
Spicy green beans, Heartplan, 132-133
Splurging, 102
Stanford heart disease study, 23-26
Steak, 112
Stouffer hotel chain, 115
Strangers, interacting with, 91-92
Streptokinase, 198
Stress, xi, 31-52
  atherosclerosis and, 8
  and blood pressure measurement, 27-28
  chronic, 93-95
  defined, 33-36
  drug therapy for, 161-162
  emotional entrapment and, xii, 42-46, 48-49, 78-86
  as emphasis of post-heart attack group sessions, 163-165
  "hot" reactors to, 28, 35-36, 95
  hypertension and, 17
  job-related, 16, 17, 92-93, 100
  from major life changes, 49-52, 93, 94, 96
  from minor irritants, 93, 95-101

Stress *(cont.)*:
  banking, 96-97
  commuting, 93, 97-98
  doctor appointments, 98
  general strategies for, 99-101
  shopping, 97
  vacations, 98-99
  physiological responses to, 27-28, 31-33, 36, 145-146
  positive vs. negative, 33-34
  reduction of, in Heartplan, 92-101, 145-149
  relaxation techniques for, 95, 145-149
  and risk of cardiovascular disease, 16, 21-23, 31-52
  Sisyphus syndrome and, xii, 37-42, 48-49
  sudden death from, 32
  thresholds for, 93
  type A behavior and, xi-xii, 46-49, 86-92
Stress test, exercise, 11, 141, 171, 184, 185
Strokes:
  aspirin for prevention of, 29
  diabetics at risk for, 16
  family history of, 16
  as first symptoms of cardiovascular disease, 10
Stuffed peppers, Heartplan, 132
Sumerian civilization, heart as viewed by, 3
Supermarkets, minor irritants at, 97
Surgery, 183-194
  artifical heart implantation, 193-194
  coronary angioplasty, 186-188
  coronary bypass, 50, 62, 63, 65, 149-150, 183-190
  emotional aspects of, 190-191
  heart transplantation, 191-192, 198
  recovery from, 190-191
Sushi, 113
Swimming, 143, 144, 174

Sympathetic nervous system, 31, 160
Systolic pressure, 6, 24, 25

Tar, 28
Target zone, 139, 140
Television repairers, 99
Tenormin, 160
Tex-Mex cuisine, 113–114, 131–132
Thallium scans, 11–12
Thoreau, Henry David, 42
Three-vessel disease, 8, 187
Thrombi (*see* Blood clots, arterial)
Time urgency, 46, 47, 88
  lessening of, 89–91
Timelessness, experience of, 91
Tissue plasminogen activator (TPA), 198
Tofutti, 110
Tradespeople, minor irritants from, 99
Tranquilizers, 58, 161–162
Transplants, heart, 191–192, 198
Trans-telephonic monitoring (TTM), 13
Triglycerides, 18, 20, 29, 161
Type A behavior, xi–xii, 46–48
  characteristics of, 47, 88
  modification of, 86–92
    counseling for, 88, 89
    and lessening of hostility, 91–92
    and lessening of time urgency, 89–91
    motivation in, 89
    in post-heart attack group sessions, 164
  personality type independent of, 86–87
  Sisyphus syndrome and emotional entrapment combined with, 48–49
  success and, 86, 87
Type A Behavior and Your Heart (Friedman and Rosenman), 88
Type B behavior, 46, 47

Unemployment, 96

Vacations, 98–99
Valium, 162
Vegetable dishes, Heartplan:
  coleslaw, 132
  eggplant spread, 134
  gazpacho, 131
  German-style potato salad, 132
  Italian vegetable casserole, 133
  marinara sauce, 135–136
  spicy green beans, 132–133
  stuffed peppers, 132
  vegetarian chili, 131–132
  wild rice with mushrooms, 131
Veins, 6
  saphenous, 183

Walking, 143, 174
  race-, 144
Warm-up exercises, 138–139
Watches, learning to do without, 91
Weight reduction:
  hypertension controlled with, 18, 161, 178–179
  pace of, 102
  (*See also* Obesity)
Weight Watchers, 165
Westin hotel chain, 115
Wild rice with mushrooms, Heartplan, 131
Winston, Mary, 136
Wolf, Stuart, 37
Women:
  cardiovascular disease in, 16
  cigarette smoking by, 20, 25
  HDL levels in, 19
  oral contraceptives taken by, 20, 25, 28
  RISKO assessment for, 25–26
  Sisyphus syndrome in, 38–39
Worcestershire sauce, 110
Workaholics, 38, 71–73

Workplace:
  commuting to, 93, 97–98
  obvious entrapment at, 79–81
  returning to, after heart attack, 62–64, 164
  role of, in setting new priorities and realistic goals, 75–78

Workplace *(cont.)*:
  stress associated with, 16, 17, 92–93, 100

Xanax, 162
Xenografts, 191–192, 198

Yogurt, 103